Exchange Politics

Exchange Politics

Opposing Obamacare in Battleground States

David K. Jones

OXFORD
UNIVERSITY PRESS

OXFORD
UNIVERSITY PRESS

Oxford University Press is a department of the University of Oxford. It furthers the University's objective of excellence in research, scholarship, and education by publishing worldwide. Oxford is a registered trade mark of Oxford University Press in the UK and certain other countries.

Published in the United States of America by Oxford University Press
198 Madison Avenue, New York, NY 10016, United States of America.

CIP data is on file at the Library of Congress
ISBN 978-0-19-067724-4 (pbk.)
ISBN 978-0-19-067723-7 (hbk.)

For Sarah, Olivia, Anne, and Thomas

CONTENTS

PREFACE AND ACKNOWLEDGMENTS

This was a fun book to write. I did much of the research in real time, as state and federal leaders struggled over what to do about health insurance exchanges. My first interview was in Lansing, Michigan, in the summer of 2011. At that point the Supreme Court had not yet announced they would consider the lawsuit filed by 26 states against the constitutionality of the Affordable Care Act (ACA). It was far from certain that President Barack Obama would be reelected the next year and remain in a position to continuing implementing the reform. It was also 4 years before the Supreme Court would consider *King v. Burwell* and 5 years before Donald Trump would be elected president.

The more than 200 interviews with state and federal leaders between June 2011 and September 2016 (with follow-up conversations in early 2017) gave me a front row seat to the intergovernmental drama surrounding health insurance exchanges and the ACA. I watched each of these major events with great interest not only for the policy outcomes but also for what it would mean for my research. I would have had to go in a vastly different direction if the Supreme Court had struck down the entire law in 2012, for example.

As daunting as it was to write a dissertation about events as they were happening, it gave me unique opportunities that might not otherwise have been available to a doctoral student. These include being lead author on commentary articles in places like the *New England Journal of Medicine* and the *Journal of the American Medical Association*, and on an op-ed in the *Washington Post*. I enjoyed speaking with reporters, talking to physician groups, and testifying before the Michigan House Health Policy Committee in January 2012 about my research to that point.

There are many people I would like to thank who helped make this book possible. First and foremost I thank my dissertation committee at the University of Michigan. Scott Greer was a fantastic advisor and committee chair who believed in the work I was doing and regularly made it better.

I am incredibly grateful to Peter Jacobson, Helen Levy, and Barry Rabe for their contributions and mentorship.

The University of Michigan was an incredible place to study health policy. There are too many professors in the School of Public Health and the Department of Political Science for me to name them all, but I would like to give special thanks to two people who became valued collaborators and mentors: John Ayanian and Nicholas Bagley. Thank you also to Marianne Udow-Phillips and others at the nearby Center for Healthcare Research & Transformation (CHRT) for your collaboration and feedback.

The many friends I made at Michigan provided invaluable emotional support, listened to presentations, and read various iterations of this work. I am particularly grateful for collaborations with Kate Bradley, Heather Elliott, and Phil Singer. Eddie Miller, Sarah Gollust, and Pamela McCann provided invaluable guidance on how to navigate a doctorate at Michigan and then on life as an assistant professor.

I am grateful to many scholars outside the University of Michigan who provided important support and insight along the way. In particular I thank Jonathan Oberlander of the University of North Carolina, who, despite cheering for all the wrong sports teams, has been a fantastic mentor and friend. Many others at Carolina have provided invaluable support since I completed a master's of science in public health there in 2009. I also thank Colleen Grogan of the University of Chicago and former editor of the *Journal of Health Politics, Policy, and Law* (JHPPL) for her collaboration and mentorship. This group, along with those participating in the health politics section of the American Political Science Association, has been an incredible source of ideas and encouragement.

Thank you to the many mentors, colleagues, and friends at Boston University who have been extremely supportive, particularly David Rosenbloom, who was the chair who hired me and regularly encouraged me throughout the publication of this book. Thank you to the Robert Wood Johnson Foundation's Health Policy Scholars, for whom I had the privilege of being a research assistant at the University of Michigan. Special thanks to the five undergraduate students who provided research assistance to me over the course of 3 years through the University of Michigan's Undergraduate Research Opportunities Program (UROP): Alex Coburn and Sahil Gosain (2011–2012), Alex Bernard and Hannah Mesa (2012–2013), and Alexa Abbott (2013–2014).

I give particular thanks to Margaret Henbest and John Rusche, who were both members of the Idaho House Health and Welfare Committee when I was an intern in the Idaho Legislature during the 2006 legislative session. It was in Boise that I gained a deep interest in state politics and federalism. My fascination with health policymaking and intergovernmental relations grew tremendously during an internship later that year with the Honourable Rob Merrifield, who at the time was Chair of the Health Committee in the Canadian House of Commons. These interests were strengthened while working with Pam Silberman and everyone else at the North Carolina Institute of Medicine and have continued to grow with support from mentors such as Chris Koller of the Millbank Memorial Fund.

I am honored that the thesis this manuscript emerged from was given the Outstanding Dissertation Award by AcademyHealth. I am grateful for funding received from a variety of sources, including grants and fellowships from the Rackham Graduate School at the University of Michigan, the Blue Cross Blue Shield of Michigan Foundation Student Research Award, the Agency for Healthcare Research and Quality doctoral traineeship, the Martha and Ernest Hammel Award, the Jim Bernstein Health Policy Fellowship, the Jean Monnet Fellowship, and grants from the Department of Health Management and Policy at the University of Michigan.

I thank the many people I interviewed for this project. This book truly would not have been possible without them. I also thank David McBride at Oxford University Press and the two anonymous reviewers whose feedback helped me improve the manuscript.

Most importantly, I thank my family. My parents, Debra Bingham and Jeffrey Jones, along with my stepfather Kent Hamilton, are a constant source of support, inspiration, and love. I am grateful for my amazingly devoted grandparents and extended family. I am pleased to dedicate this work to my children Olivia, Anne, and Thomas, all of whom were born while I was in graduate school. They bring so much joy into my life. My wife, Sarah Sacuto, is a wonderful partner and friend. I cannot adequately express my gratitude for her support.

Exchange Politics

CHAPTER 1

Introduction

The Patient Protection and Affordable Care Act of 2010 (PPACA or ACA) is the most significant health reform legislation enacted in generations and is the signature policy achievement of the Obama presidency. Presidents since at least Harry Truman had tried and failed to pass comprehensive health reform. This was a hard-fought victory for President Obama and his congressional allies, particularly since not a single Republican voted for the final bill in either the House of Representatives or the Senate.

The ACA is a complex law made of up 10 titles, each with numerous sections. The core of the reform is an expansion of coverage to millions of Americans who previously did not fit into an existing program. The law mandates that everyone be covered and creates new ways to make this possible for people who previously could not afford insurance. Children are now allowed to stay on their parents' plan until the age of twenty-six. Insurers can no longer deny benefits because of preexisting conditions. Companies with fifty or more full-time employees are required to offer affordable health insurance or pay a fine. Medicaid is expanded to cover anyone poor enough to qualify, not just people in specific categories, such as children, pregnant women, and parents. People who are not poor enough to qualify for Medicaid but are not well enough off to be able to afford insurance can receive government subsidies to purchase private plans using an online marketplace called an exchange.

This was not the liberal dream of a single-payer system, but it was nonetheless the largest expansion of insurance coverage in the United States since the creation of Medicare and Medicaid in 1965. Its passage was the culmination of decades of incremental reforms, an intense presidential campaign, and two years of Capitol Hill maneuvering (McDonough 2011, Starr 2011). Democrats were disappointed this was the best they could get, but thrilled and relieved to finally pass a major health reform law.

President Obama celebrated this accomplishment before jubilant crowds at two bill-signing ceremonies on March 23, 2010. In the East Room of the White House he declared, "Today, after almost a century of trying; today, after over a year of debate; today, after all the votes have been tallied—health insurance reform becomes the law of the land in the United States of America." Later that day he told a group of doctors, nurses, and patients, "health care reform is no longer an unmet promise. It is the law of the land. It is the law of the land" (White House 2010). Senator Max Baucus, who had played a key role as chair of the Senate Finance Committee similarly declared, "Now it is a fact. Now it is law. Now it is history."

Despite these grand claims of success, the fight over health reform was far from over. Supporters of health reform learned that enacting a statute is not enough to produce meaningful change and that politics does not end once a bill becomes a law (Pressman and Wildavsky 1979, Patashnik 2008). Countless decisions needed to be made and billions of dollars spent before major elements of the reform would fully go into effect and people would start receiving insurance benefits. The ACA remained vulnerable long after it was enacted.

National opponents used a multipronged strategy to disrupt implementation of the law they nicknamed Obamacare. They focused on winning elections, filing lawsuits, and passing laws to undermine the reform. The ultimate goal was to repeal the ACA, but at the very least they hoped to discourage proponents of the reform and frustrate planning.

It would be two and a half years before Speaker of the US House of Representatives John Boehner (R-OH) eventually conceded that the ACA is indeed "the law of the land" (Nather 2012)—but only after more than thirty congressional attempts at repeal, a 5–4 decision by the US Supreme Court, and President Obama's reelection in 2012. Even after Boehner's concession, the reform would need to survive another two dozen repeal votes in the House, more legal challenges, a repeal bill vetoed by President Obama in early 2016, and the threat that future elections would embolden and empower Republicans hell-bent on repeal.

Donald Trump's election in November 2016 put the fight over health reform into a state of chaos. Republicans are now in a position to undo major portions of the ACA, if not the whole law. Whether they will follow through with their seven years' worth of threats is yet to be seen as I write this. The Republican takeover of government in 2017 is the culmination of a determined strategy largely focused on challenging and undermining Obamacare. Understanding what happened during the years immediately after the ACA's enactment will be crucial to understanding whatever comes next.

ACCIDENTAL FEDERALISM

A remarkable aspect of this story is that many of the most consequential and dramatic fights over the ACA's implementation took place not in Washington, DC, but in state capitals around the country. States were given an important role in developing health insurance exchanges, reviewing premium increases, and enforcing new market regulations (Greer 2011; Béland, Rocco, and Waddan 2014). States would ultimately gain even greater prominence in defining the required benefits of plans sold on the exchange and deciding whether to accept or reject the Medicaid expansion.

Shepherding the implementation of federal law through fifty separate states would have been an enormous challenge for the Obama administration under ideal political conditions. An implementation period spanning three election cycles (2010, 2012, and 2014) left the reform vulnerable to political opposition and partisan shifts in control, amplifying the challenge of implementation. Many supporters therefore considered the ACA "an uneasy victory" (Starr 2011) because the most comprehensive federal health reform enacted in generations was to a large extent placed in the hands of state-level leaders who fervently opposed the law's very existence.

Conservative state leaders took their cues from congressional Republicans and used the same obstructionist strategies of winning elections, passing—or in many cases blocking—legislation, and filing lawsuits. For example, within minutes of President Obama's bill signing ceremony, the attorney general of Florida held a press conference announcing a lawsuit against the ACA's constitutionality. The number of states signing on eventually grew to 26. In June 2012 the Supreme Court sided with the Obama administration on the individual mandate, but the ruling making Medicaid expansion optional opened up a new front in the intergovernmental battle over health reform. Meanwhile another lawsuit—ultimately reaching the Supreme Court as *King v. Burwell*—was filed arguing that the ACA's wording meant that consumers in states without a state-run exchange were ineligible to receive government assistance to purchase insurance. The Obama administration won that case as well, but opponents hoped that if enough states resisted the exchanges and Medicaid, the law would be ineffective and collapse under its own weight, embarrassing Democrats and making the ACA's repeal inevitable.

Why did the writers of the ACA allow the reform to be vulnerable by giving states such a prominent role in its implementation? Although Republican governors and other leaders were expected to make a lot of noise complaining about the law, the Obama administration, scholars, and reporters believed most would ultimately comply. This was a gross miscalculation, but seemed reasonable in 2010 because state leaders regularly say they want as much flexibility as possible. States had the opportunity to use federal money to make major changes, while at the same time claiming credit for everything that worked and blaming the Obama administration for anything that did not. Fox and Markel (2010) cited historical examples to suggest that although implementation is hard, "antagonism has a half-life."

The ACA's intergovernmental compromise was born more out of political necessity than a true consensus over the appropriate balance between levels of government. Federalism debates were frequently invoked during the congressional battle over health reform, particularly in conversations about how to reconcile the differences between the House and Senate versions. Supporters of the House bill argued that a national health insurance exchange would be more effective because of greater bargaining power and lower administrative costs (Jost 2009). Rather than require that fifty states do the work of developing essentially identical information technology (IT) software and then spend the resources to manage an exchange, they believed it would be more efficient to have a single exchange developed by the national government.

Many Senate Democrats countered that the national exchange concentrated too much power in Washington at the expense of states. Senator Nelson warned, "the national exchange is unnecessary and I wouldn't support something that would start us down the road of federal regulation of insurance and a single-payer plan" (Budoff Brown 2010). Supporters of the Senate bill also argued that by running their own exchange, states could determine how it interacts with their state's Medicaid program, define the role of brokers and agents, and tailor outreach efforts to local conditions (Interviews 2011–2013). The Senate version ultimately did not contain a public option, or a government-run insurance plan against which private companies would have to compete (Hacker 2008, 2009). Instead, the Senate version contained a threat that the federal government would step in to create an exchange in any state that refused to do it on their own.

In early negotiations between the two chambers to combine their respective bills, President Obama initially supported the House version with a national exchange (Werner 2010). However, Ted Kennedy's death in August 2009 and Scott Brown's surprise victory in the Massachusetts special election the following January reduced the Democrats' total in the Senate from 60 to 59 seats. Although still a formidable majority, they no longer had enough seats to overcome a Republican filibuster.

Democrats were split on how to respond, with some such as White House Chief of Staff Rahm Emmanuel calling for Democrats to retreat and aim for a more incremental bill. Others, such as Nancy Pelosi (D-CA) and Harry Reid (D-NV) convinced President Obama to follow through with the more comprehensive reform (Budoff Brown and Thrush 2010). To do this, Senate Democrats passed the ACA using a budget reconciliation process requiring a simple fifty-one-vote majority. Their improvised approach only worked if House Democrats voted for the Senate's bill without amendments and without the opportunity to negotiate in a conference committee. The version of reform favoring state flexibility—and therefore opening the door to state-led resistance—thus became law by default.

HEALTH INSURANCE EXCHANGES

Health insurance exchanges were a centerpiece of the reform and the primary front in the intergovernmental battle over the ACA's implementation, at least until the Supreme Court ruling in 2012 made the Medicaid expansion optional. An exchange is a website where consumers can shop for health insurance, comparing plans side by side, analogous to buying airline tickets on Travelocity.com. They are the mechanism through which people with qualifying incomes receive federal subsidies to reduce the costs of premiums.

Scholars and reporters warned that establishing state-level exchanges would not be easy. Dozens of difficult decisions would have to be made, including how intensely to regulate plans, whether representatives of insurance companies can sit on the board of directors, and whether to house the exchange within a government agency or establish an independent entity. *Time Magazine* (Tumulty, Pickert, and Park 2010) called setting up an exchange "the most important challenge for the states" and quoted Oregon's governor saying, "I wake up worrying how I'm going to get from 2010 to 2014" when people would start receiving benefits through the exchange. But the major challenges described were developing the IT, having enough insurance plans to facilitate robust competition, and convincing enough consumers to sign up. The obstacle was not expected to be convincing states to participate.

The health insurance exchange was a part of the ACA initially expected to elude controversy and attract bipartisan support. Supporters of an exchange hoped the idea would draw political strength from a flexible identity as "conservative means to liberal ends" (Jones, Bradley, and Oberlander 2014). Progressives would like the expansion of coverage, and conservatives would like that the expansion comes through a state-based market-oriented mechanism in which private insurers compete. The potential for bipartisan political appeal is evident in polling data. In a June 2010 Kaiser Family Foundation survey, 87% of all respondents—including 77% of Republicans—said they had a very or somewhat favorable opinion of exchanges, the highest level of support for any feature of the ACA (KFF 2010).

The ACA's exchanges were largely modeled on purchasing pools supported by Republicans since the 1990s, most notably the creation of the Massachusetts Health Connector (Jones, Oberlander, and Bradley 2014). The 2006 Massachusetts reform enjoyed strong bipartisan support from Democrats, the state's Republican governor (Mitt Romney), and GOP legislators. The law passed the state House and Senate by a nearly unanimous vote (McDonough et al. 2006), providing Democrats with both policy and political blueprints for passing health reform.

Prominent conservatives supported the concept of state-based insurance exchanges in the run-up to the ACA's passage. Edmund Haislmaier (2006) of the Heritage Foundation praised the Massachusetts reform saying that governors and legislators would be "well advised to consider this basic model as a framework for health care reform in their own states." Republican governors in places such as Mississippi and Utah were following Mitt Romney's lead in developing insurance exchanges. Marketplace organizers similar to the Connector remained a part of GOP alternatives during the intensely partisan congressional debate over the ACA. For example, the 2009 Patients' Choice Act, cosponsored by Senator Tom Coburn (Oklahoma) and Congressman Paul Ryan (Wisconsin)—subsequently Mitt Romney's running mate in the 2012 presidential election and Speaker of the House beginning in 2015—proposed creating state exchanges that would provide a "one-stop marketplace for health insurance" (Ryan 2009, Coburn 2013).

Supporters of the ACA may have preferred a single national exchange, but now needed to promote federalism (Jones, Bradley, and Oberander 2014). Whether to provide credibility to the threat of preemption or because they thought most states would comply, the writers of the law did not give the federal government money to set up exchanges on behalf of states. Instead, the administration used both carrots and sticks to try to induce cooperation. The Department of Health and Human Services (HHS) was willing to write essentially blank checks to state leaders through planning and establishment grants.[1] Conservative leaders were reluctant to be seen as partners with the Obama administration, but feared that by refusing to comply with this part of the law they would actually be giving greater control to the Obama administration over the insurance market in their state. Prominent interest groups such as hospitals, insurers, providers, and consumers had a strong preference for local control and were expected to pressure their leaders accordingly. Given this combination of money, pressure, and threats, there was a strong expectation among interest groups and within the Obama administration that virtually every state would choose to establish their own exchange.

Yet by the time open enrollment for coverage on the exchanges began in October 2013, only 16 states (and the District of Columbia) had chosen to create their own exchange. This is a stunning outcome and was a huge disappointment for the Obama administration. It refused to believe states would resist to the point of ceding control to the federal government and so was thoroughly unprepared for the task of opening 34 exchanges. HHS had to raid the Prevention Fund and other parts of the agency to come up with money to do this work (Harkin 2013). This contributed to, along with bad choices in selecting vendors to develop the IT, a disastrous rollout of healthcare.gov, the website for the federal government's exchanges in resistant states.

Why did so few states choose to create an exchange? What does this mean for the success of the ACA, and what does it tell us about American federalism? This book sets out to answer these questions. This story takes us to state houses across the country to witness the seemingly minor but highly consequential differences in how states make decisions. This includes tracking procedural details such as how often and in what time of year a legislature meets, whether it has term limits, and whether insurance commissioners are appointed or independently elected.

The debate over health insurance exchanges mirrored—and to a large extent fueled—the rise and growing power of the Tea Party at the local level. In many states the Tea Party was a divisive force on the right, foreshadowing the growing divide within the national Republican Party that would ultimately topple House Speaker John Boehner and lead to Donald Trump winning the 2016 nomination and election. Democrats grossly misjudged how state leaders would react to the exchanges, and watched helplessly as the ACA's reliance on states—which was supposed to be a major selling point to skeptical conservatives—nearly led to its unraveling. Depending on what happens in 2017 and beyond, it may yet still.

Understanding how states made these decisions is crucial to understanding whether health insurance exchanges around the country are succeeding or failing. Opponents of the ACA highlight the growing number of counties where only one insurance company is selling plans, undermining the premise of an exchange that competition will bring prices down. The stories in this book suggest that state-level Republicans may be to blame for the failure of exchanges as much as—or more than—the Democrats who wrote and passed the law.

MORE THAN PARTISANSHIP

Partisanship, the notion that Republicans refused to support an idea because it was endorsed by President Obama and other Democrats, is one of the most common explanations for why so many states rejected creating a health insurance exchange (Young 2012, Burke and Kamarck 2013, Purdum 2013, Rigby and Haselwerdt 2013). The final breakdown of state decision-making supports the argument that partisan patterns explain which states rejected or created an exchange: of the 30 Republican governors in office when the exchanges opened in October 2013, only three (10%) presided over the creation of a state-based exchange, compared to 13 of the 20 Democratic governors (65%).[2] Republicans controlled at least one chamber in four of the remaining seven states led by a Democrat.

Partisanship is a particularly compelling explanation for the states that made the decision quickly. Jones, Bradley, and Oberlander (2014) chart the evolution of the Republican response between 2010 and 2013. Nearly every state initially hedged bets, with all but Alaska and Minnesota accepting $1 million grants to begin planning, including most states that were part of the Florida-led lawsuit. The partisan landscape changed dramatically after the 2010 midterm elections, and newly elected Republican governors began to give back grants accepted by their predecessors. In some cases—such as Sam Brownback in Kansas, Mary Fallin in Oklahoma, and Scott Walker in Wisconsin—Republican governors returned grants that they had defended accepting just months earlier.

By November 2011, when the US Supreme Court announced it would hear the case against the ACA's constitutionality, only twelve state legislatures had passed a bill creating an exchange and one governor had done so by executive order. More than half of these early adopters were led entirely by Democrats, with Schwarzenegger (CA) and Brian Sandoval (NV) being the only Republican governors to have signed legislation creating an exchange since the ACA's enactment. At the same time, fourteen states had already committed to not creating an exchange. Republicans controlled twenty-five of these twenty-eight legislative chambers, and all but three of these states were led by Republican governors.

However, partisanship is an incomplete explanation obscuring important aspects of how states made their decisions, how far many states went in their consideration of an exchange, and Republican infighting over the issue. This is particularly true for the remaining 23 states that were undecided as of November 2011. Although 16 of these states were led by Republican governors (see Table 1.1), they accepted an average of $20 million in federal grants by November 2011 to actively study and plan for the creation of an exchange (Kaiser Family Foundation [KFF] 2014b).

The Obama administration worked hard to convince as many of these states to step up as possible. In addition to giving out money, deadlines were extended multiple times and the wording to describe the balance of power between levels of government constantly evolved to signal greater state flexibility. By mid-2012 states could choose a "partnership" exchange in which they retain some control even though they were using the federal website.

Many state-level Republicans hoped the decision would disappear, either because the Supreme Court would strike down the whole law or Mitt Romney would defeat President Obama and follow through on his

Table 1.1. STATE DECISION-MAKING AND PARTISAN CONTROL, AS OF NOVEMBER 2011

	Unified R Control	Mixed Control, R Governor	Unified D Control	Mixed Control, D Governor
Exchange	UT	NV	CA,[a] CT, HI, MA, MD, RI,[b] VT, WA, WV	CO, OR
Undecided	AL, AZ, ID, IN, NE,[c] PA, SD, TN, WI	IA, ME, MI, MS, NJ, NM, VA	DE, IL	KY, MN, MO, NY, NC
No Exchange	AR, FL, GA, KS, LA, ND, OH, OK, SC, TX, WY	AK		MT, NH

[a] Legislation creating an exchange was signed into law in 2010 by Republican Arnold Schwarzenegger, though by November 2011 the state was led by Democrat Jerry Brown.
[b] Governor Lincoln Chafee had been a Republican while in the U.S. Senate, was independent when elected governor, but subsequently joined the Democratic Party.
[c] Nebraska's legislature is officially non-partisan.

promises to dismantle the ACA. When neither happened, just five of these twenty-three states decided to create a state-based exchange. Only two of the sixteen of these states led by Republican governors opted for maintaining control. However, simply attributing state decisions to partisanship misses the level of internal conflict in many of these states. In many cases, the most important division in these states was among Republicans, not between Republicans and Democrats. The fight over exchanges was part of a larger battle for the soul of the Republican Party.

Roll call data is evidence that many Republican leaders across the country were at least initially willing to support creating a health insurance exchange in their state (Jones, Bradley, and Oberlander 2014). In the three years after the ACA's passage in March 2010, floor votes were held on twenty-seven exchange bills in at least one chamber of twenty-two states[3] (see Table 1.2). More than sixty bills to establish an exchange were introduced in other states but never received a floor vote (CBPP 2013). There are clear partisan differences in these votes, but Republicans were hardly unanimous in their opposition. On these bills, 91% of Democratic legislators voted in favor of legislation creating an exchange, compared to 42% of Republican legislators.

Less talked about by scholars and pundits, it was surprising that Democrats were so united in favor of state-level exchanges. Nearly 90% voted in favor in the states that considered legislation. In the early stages of implementation Democrats were worried that the entire ACA might be eliminated by the Supreme Court or by a new president in 2013. Creating a state-level exchange before then was a way to entrench a core component of the law while also undermining the lawsuit. But Democrats remained supportive beyond 2012, even as it became clear that the type of exchange that might be created would be weaker and less regulated than what they preferred. They could have bypassed Republican state leaders they did not trust in order to default to the Obama administration, whose policy preferences more closely matched theirs. When asked about this tension, they explained that they genuinely thought state control would be better.

The split among Republicans over the exchanges can largely be traced to the growth of the Tea Party after Rick Santelli's CNBC rant in February 2009 (Santelli 2009). Tea Party activists became the guerrilla warriors in the fight against Obamacare. They would eventually insert themselves into the minutiae of legislative politics and government contracting. But their first focus was winning elections by defeating Democrats and Republicans they felt were too moderate. They were a major force in the dramatic rightward shift across the country in November 2010. Republicans made extraordinary gains and reclaimed a majority in the US

Table 1.2. ROLL CALL OF FLOOR VOTES ON LEGISLATION TO CREATE EXCHANGES, 2006–2013

Pre-ACA

State	Date	Legislature (upper-lower)	Bill	Status	% R	% D
MA	April 2006	D-D	Ch. 58	Enacted	91.3%	100.0%
UT	March 2009	R-R	HB 188	Enacted	93.9%	96.3%
				Total	92.6%	98.1%

Post-ACA

State	Date	Legislature (upper-lower)	Bill	Status	% R	% D
CA[a]	Sept 2010	D-D	SB 900	Enacted	2.4%	94.6%
CA[a]	Sept 2010	D-D	AB 1602	Enacted	4.8%	93.2%
MS[b]	March 2011	D-R	HB 1220	Passed, not law	59.8%	91.1%
WV	April 2011	D-D	SB408	Enacted	0.0%	97.8%
RI	April 2011	D-D	SB 87	Passed, not law	85.7%	80.0%
NM	April 2011	D-D	SB 38	Vetoed	21.3%	92.3%
MD	April 2011	D-D	HB166	Enacted	41.1%	94.7%
MO	April 2011	R-R	SB 609	Passed House	97.2%	96.4%
VA[c]	April 2011	D-R	HB 2434	Enacted	92.0%	35.6%
WA	May 2011	D-D	SB5445	Enacted	33.8%	97.6%
NC	May 2011	R-R	HB 115	Passed House	95.6%	34.6%
VT	May 2011	D-D	HB202	Enacted	0.0%	90.4%
CO	June 2011	D-R	SB11-200	Enacted	27.1%	98.1%
NJ	June 2011	D-D	A1930	Passed Assembly	0.0%	80.8%
NV	June 2011	D-D	SB440	Enacted	88.9%	97.2%
OR	June 2011	D-S	SB99	Enacted	63.6%	95.7%
CT	July 2011	D-D	SB 921	Enacted	25.8%	94.2%
HI	July 2011	D-D	SB1348	Enacted	89.0%	100.0%
ND	Nov 2011	R-R	HB 1474	Failed House	14.5%	87.0%
MI	Nov 2011	R-R	SB 693	Passed Senate	50.0%	100.0%
AL	April 2012	R-R	HB 245	Passed House	92.4%	79.5%
NJ	May 2012	D-D	A2171/ S 1319	Vetoed	0.0%	87.5%
NJ	Dec 2012	D-D	A3186/S2135	Vetoed	0.0%	89.0%
NM	Feb 2013	D-D	HB 168	Failed House	0.0%	79.0%
MN	March 2013	D-D	HF 5	Enacted	3.0%	96.0%
NM	March 2013	D-D	SB 221	Enacted	96.0%	84.0%
ID	March 2013	R-R	HB 248	Enacted	53.0%	95.0%
				Total	42.1%	87.5%

[a] Two companion bills were enacted the same day.
[b] Bill did not make it through a conference committee.
[c] Bill states intent to create an exchange, but does not authorize any particular action.

House of Representatives, while significantly narrowing the Democrats' margin in the Senate. The GOP enjoyed a net gain of six governors, twelve lower houses, and seven upper houses. When these leaders took office in January 2011, twenty-nine states had Republican governors (in addition to a Republican-turned-Independent governor in Rhode Island), and twenty-one had unified governments with the GOP also controlling both legislative chambers. Republicans enjoyed strong majorities in the chambers they controlled, with an average margin of thirty-three in lower houses and thirteen in upper houses (NCSL 2011). Republican incumbents felt pressure to be more conservative to avoid a primary challenge. Blue and purple states turned red, while red states got redder. The partisan shift to the right complicated state-level implementation of exchanges, though not always in predictable ways.

EXCHANGE POLITICS

This book takes an in-depth look at the fight over health insurance exchanges in four states: Idaho, Michigan, Mississippi, and New Mexico. Decision-making took many twists in these states, including governors vetoing authorizing legislation before eventually supporting an exchange, Republicans disagreeing strongly with each other, and Democrats unsure of how to react. Legislation to create an exchange passed in seven of the eight legislative chambers, yet was enacted only in Idaho and New Mexico. Even then, they decided so late in the process that they had to ultimately rely on the federal website for at least the first year.

Each of these states was among the twenty-three that remained undecided as of November 2011. Although focusing on this group does not allow for a complete look at the greater role that partisanship seemed to play in the twenty-seven states (plus the District of Columbia) that quickly accepted or rejected an exchange, this allows for a clearer understanding of the interactions between partisanship, state politics, and federalism. These twenty-three states remained up for grabs the longest and were those the Obama administration was trying hardest to convince. Idaho and New Mexico were two of the very last states to choose to create an exchange, whereas Michigan and Mississippi were two of the states that came closest but did not. Examining the similarities and differences between these four states on either side of this decision sheds light on the factors that affected how the rest of this group responded.

All four of these states were led by Republican governors but differed in partisan control of the legislature. Both the upper and lower chambers were controlled by Republicans in Idaho and Michigan, by Democrats in New Mexico, and switched from mixed control to Republican control during the period of analysis in Mississippi. Michigan and New Mexico voted for Barack Obama in 2008 and 2012, whereas Idaho and Mississippi voted for John McCain and Mitt Romney (see Table 1.3). The states also vary in other important ways, including whether they have legislative term limits, a year-round legislature, and an elected insurance commissioner.

I focus on the period between March 2010 when the ACA was signed into law and the start of the first open enrollment in October 2013. This was when the key decisions were made. A lot of important events took place before and after this period. In many cases the roots of the debate in a state go back at least a decade; in every case, the struggle over creating exchanges extends well beyond 2013. This book cannot therefore be a complete evaluation of all the factors that caused an exchange to succeed or fail. It is still too soon to tell.

The ascendency of Donald Trump and the threat of changes to the ACA make it far more important—not less—to understand how states responded to the ACA between 2010 and 2014. Every state will experience changes to the ACA differently according to what changes they have adopted during this period as a result of the ACA. The practical impact

Table 1.3. SUMMARY OF CASE STUDY STATES

	Idaho	Michigan	Mississippi	New Mexico
Governor	R	R	R	R
House	R	R	R	D
Senate	R	R	R	D
2012 Election	Romney	Obama	Romney	Obama
Exchange	State	Federal	Federal	State
Joined lawsuit	Yes	Yes	Yes	No
Bureaucratic capacity	16th	1st	40th	30th
Term limits	No	Yes	No	No
Year-round legislature	No	Yes	No	No
Planning grant	$1m	$1m	$1m	$1m
Early innovator grant	–	–	–	–
Level 1 est. grant	$20.4	$40.6	$20.1	$34.3
Elected ins. comm.	No	No	Yes	No
# Insurers >5% market	4	4	4	2
Market share of largest insurer	38%	59%	54%	59%
Uninsured rate	18%	13%	19%	21%

of any subsequent changes will largely be determined by whether a state expanded Medicaid and adopted its own health insurance exchange.

I find that four key factors shaped how states responded to the dilemma of whether or not to create a health insurance exchange (see Table 1.4): first, governors were the most important individuals in each state's debate. However, although gubernatorial support was a necessary condition, it was not sufficient for the creation of a state-based exchange. Some Republican governors supported state control of an exchange but were unable to convince their legislature to cooperate with the Obama administration.

Second, the Tea Party was an amazingly successful counterweight to organized interest groups, particularly given its lack of clear organization. National groups such as Americans for Prosperity, Right to Life, the Cato Institute, and the American Legislative Exchange Council (ALEC) played a prominent role in supporting Tea Party opposition, as did their sister organizations at the state level. They believed they could topple the entire law if enough states resisted the health insurance exchanges. ALEC published *The State Legislator's Guide to Repealing Obamacare* urging leaders to not apply for any exchange grants and to return any they had received (ALEC 2011). Edmund Haislmaier of the Heritage Foundation spoke at an ALEC conference in early 2011 calling for "an unrelenting fight [against Obamacare]" with "house by house, floor by floor, room by room combat," arguing, "There will be numerous places and lines of attack where we can undermine this law" (Mooney 2011).

Third, resistance could be overcome if state conditions allowed for the development of "pockets of expertise" in the legislature. These are legislators who have developed a high level of knowledge and influence on a particular policy issue (Burns et al. 2008). Decision-making over health

Table 1.4. INFLUENCE OF KEY ACTORS ON HEALTH INSURANCE EXCHANGE DECISION

	Gov Support 2011	Weak Tea Party	Gov Maintains Support 2012/ 2013	Strong Industry Coalition	Pockets of expertise	Exchange
Michigan	x		x	x		
Mississippi	x			x		
Idaho	x		x	x	x	x
New Mexico	x	x	x	x	x	x

insurance exchanges was relatively fragmented (Béland, Rocco, and Waddan 2016), meaning that seemingly benign differences in how state institutions are designed and operate—such as whether there are term limits—played a major role in shaping who was empowered to make decisions. One of the most important of these was timing. States experienced their role in the ACA's implementation and their interactions with the federal government differently depending on when their legislature met. For example, few states were in session much longer in 2010 after the ACA was signed into law on March 23. This amplified the importance of the 2010 elections and limited the ability of outgoing Democratic governors to entrench elements of the law before their departure. Similarly, many Republican state leaders wanted to delay making decisions on an insurance exchange until after the Supreme Court ruled on the ACA's constitutionality. Because the Supreme Court's decision in *NFIB v. Sebelius* did not come out until June 28, 2012 (NFIB v. Sebelius 2012), this meant that only the seven states with sessions extending into July could consider exchange legislation that year (Jones 2012). States have the option of holding a special session in which legislators are called back to consider specific bills. However, they vary dramatically in terms of the rules and norms of holding special sessions.

The fourth theme that emerges from these states is the importance of leadership. This is a subtle point building on what has already been said about governors and legislative experts. Borrowing a phrase from the implementation science literature, "every change needs a champion" (Bingham 2007). Whether a state moved forward on an exchange often depended on the judgment and ability of people in key positions. Anyone involved in politics and government likely understands this. But political scientists do not do a very good job of accounting for the role of individual people and tactical skill to shape outcomes. Policymakers are often treated as rational actors guided by a game theoretic calculation of incentives and payoffs. The fight over health insurance exchanges makes it clear that the judgment, preferences, and experiences of individual people are important. Yes, incentives change in response to pressure from interest groups, and actors are empowered differently as a result of the state and intergovernmental context. But within all these constraints are people making decisions. In other words, different individuals with similar incentives placed in similar circumstances might come to different conclusions about which path to take. They then possess different skills and abilities to convince others to follow.

I discuss each of themes in more depth throughout this book and in the conclusion.

LAVORATORIES OF DEMOCRACY?

All of these factors happen within the context of debates about the role of each level of government. Before turning to the first state it will be helpful to better understand the relationship between states and the federal government. American federalism is often described through baking metaphors. It is not a layered cake in which the boundaries are clearly delineated, but rather a marble cake in which the roles of each level overlap. Sometimes this overlap is cooperative, though other times it is coercive, contested, and competitive (Volden 2005, Posner 2007, Bulman-Pozen and Gerken 2009, Fox 2010, Rabe 2011). This balance varies between policies, though it can also be true at various points in the life of a single policy, as is the case with the ACA and even with the health insurance exchanges.

The fight over exchanges is a series of intergovernmental ironies. The ACA likely would not have passed had liberals been unwilling to delegate major decisions to states; however, this created an additional path to resistance for opponents. The law was supposed to be popular—or at least accepted—precisely because of its reliance on federalism. Similarly, it is ironic that the reform that came to be known as Obamacare did not reflect President Obama's preference for the House version of the reform, which included a national exchange and a mandatory Medicaid expansion (Interviews 2011–2012). Finally, opposition from state leaders lamenting what they describe as a federal takeover of the healthcare system would paradoxically pave the way for greater control by the Obama administration over insurance exchanges.

Direct state challenges to federal law have become increasingly common in recent years, with resistance to No Child Left Behind being a prominent example (McGuinn 2006, Shelly 2008, Manna 2010). Seven states filed a lawsuit against the enforcement of the Motor Voter Act of 1993 (Shelly 2008). Twenty-seven states passed a law or resolution challenging the 2005 REAL ID law, ultimately leading the federal government to extend deadlines and delay enforcement (Regan and Deering 2009). Nicholson-Crotty (2012) chronicles a history of states "leaving money on the table" by returning grants or refusing to apply for available funds. Opponents of state-based insurance exchanges regularly cited these episodes as examples of the potential power of state resistance.

There were early warnings about the difficult role that federalism would play in the ACA's implementation. Jacobs and Skocpol (2010) presciently argued, "what seemed like an obscure decision during the debate in Congress to assign extensive responsibility to states may turn out to be one of the most consequential in the future." Tim Jost (2010) similarly warned that adopting the Senate's version of reform would lead to "50 state reenactments of the battle witnessed" in Congress. In other words, before bureaucrats could do the work of actually implementing the law—such as making detailed and technical decisions about how much to ask in federal grants, how essential health benefits should be defined, which IT vendors to hire, and how extensively to regulate health insurance brokers—each state had to go through an intensely political process involving multiple branches of government.

During one of these state-level fights, the clerk of the Idaho Senate State Affairs Committee may have inadvertently suggested a new analogy for federalism and the ACA's implementation. Representative Jim Clark testified to the committee on February 17, 2010, about the Idaho Health Care Freedom Act (ID HB 391), a bill he cosponsored which would make Idaho a leader in rejecting the ACA even before it was passed. Someone asked whether this was an appropriate role for states to play while Congress was debating national policy. Representative Clark used the famous quote by Justice Brandeis about states as laboratories to suggest that states should be bold—in this case opposing the federal law. Maybe because the letter "v" is next to "b" on the keyboard, the official committee minutes record Representative Clark describing states like Idaho as "a lavatory of ideas" (ID Senate State Affairs Committee 2010). This Freudian typo hints at the discomfort of intergovernmental dynamics throughout the ACA's implementation. Federalism is messy.

Despite the added policy and political complexity, relying on states may indeed create opportunities for innovation and learning. The analogy of states as laboratories invokes images of policymakers as scientists, making informed decisions about what policies work best based on careful analysis of smaller scale experiments. Ideas can be tried out by a state before being adopted by another state or at the national level. Leaders can better predict what policy outcomes and political consequences to expect based on results elsewhere.

In many ways the ACA matches the laboratories analogy (Sparer 2011). The 2006 Massachusetts law was a major turning point in the national conversation about health reform, showing that bipartisan compromise was possible. The basic outline of the national reform (at least the coverage expansions in Titles I and II) matched the approach taken in Massachusetts: a mandate requiring everyone to be covered, high eligibility thresholds for Medicaid, and a subsidized purchasing pool to help people in the individual market purchase coverage. Many of the people who helped write the Massachusetts law played prominent roles in shaping the ACA, such as John McDonough, Jonathan Gruber, and David Cutler. Differences between states in how they implement exchanges, Medicaid expansion, rate review, and other features of the ACA can serve as natural experiments allowing policymakers and scholars to examine the differences in outcomes and make subsequent changes as a result.

But the laboratory analogy breaks down in important ways. Unlike the best scientific experiments, state-level policy is not randomized, making it difficult to predict how the results from one state will apply somewhere with a more hostile political climate or with a different policy history (Sparer and Brown 1996). States had to make important decisions about the ACA's implementation under extremely difficult time pressures, limiting how much they could really learn from each other. For example, because most states began considering running their exchange at roughly the same moment, they would likely need to make key decisions before having much evidence about which exchange models worked best and why. The final federal exchange grants expired in 2014, meaning that states waiting for more evidence would face a different decision from the states they are learning from, because they would have to establish an exchange without any federal money.

Another misleading aspect of the laboratory analogy is that states are treated as rational individuals who make policy after weighing evidence. The reality is far more complicated. Instead, states are made up of multiple factions, each competing to influence decisions. Individual stakeholders within a state may be learning from what is happening elsewhere, but that may or may not be represented in the final policy choices. This points to an important question about US federalism: when looking at the degree to which Congress delegates implementation decisions to states (Clouser McCann 2016), we should look at whether the federal statute specifies who in the state needs to act and what specific activities they need to do. Is legislation needed or can a governor act by executive order? Can an agency do things on its own and even over the opposition of its governor? The big question in many states of what to decide about whether to create an exchange ultimately came down to a battle over process and who gets to decide.

Similarly, the fight over exchanges highlights another important aspect of the laboratories metaphor: opponents of the ACA were closely watching states around the country for lessons on how to best block the reform. National organizations such as the Cato Institute and ALEC set the tone for state-level conservative think tanks and other local groups, pushing opposition over the ACA to evolve from being mostly about the individual mandate to other elements, including health insurance exchanges. One state legislator blamed these groups for what he saw as an increased nationalization of state health policy (Interview September 2016). These opponents believed the federal government was bluffing in its threat to take over state exchanges and would give in if enough states resisted. They pointed to the deadlines extensions as evidence that the Obama administration lacked the will and capacity to follow through with threats of preemption, and they challenged fellow Republicans to call the bluff. Republican legislators saw that their peers in other states were being defeated by Tea Party activists for not being aggressive enough against the ACA. This put intense pressure on Republican governors and other state leaders, who in turn became galvanized as they observed the effects of the obstructionist tactics by their counterparts elsewhere.

This episode highlights the tension between partisanship and federalism. How do Republicans—who typically prefer solutions at the local level—respond when their opposition will lead to greater federal control over a policy idea they may otherwise support? How do state-level Democrats—who typically prefer national solutions—respond when the best way to advance a policy goal is to allow for state flexibility? As will be seen throughout this book, ideology often trumps preferences for federalism (Keiser and Soss 1998; Yackee and Yackee 2009; Medoff, Dennis, and Stephens 2011; Nicholson-Crotty 2012). When it suits their ideological goals, Republicans are willing to give up control to the federal government and Democrats are willing to cede control to states.

The battle over health insurance exchanges is important not just because of the millions of people who gained access to coverage but also because of what it reveals about intergovernmental politics and the challenge of implementing a federal law at the state level. This is a dramatic and largely unprecedented instance of state leaders resisting flexibility and money to undermine a federal law they wanted repealed. Federal officials offered virtually unlimited amounts of money and made repeated threats of preemption, but seemed to be bluffing. State leaders called them on it and were offered extended deadlines, more money, and greater flexibility. Thirty-four states still rejected creating a health insurance exchange. Their resistance raises serious questions about the ability of federal leaders to induce state cooperation in other policy domains, such as education and climate change.

A Note on Methods

I use a polytheoretical approach. My goal is not to test a particular hypothesis such as that the decision was primarily driven by differences in public opinion, intergovernmental dynamics, a function of institutional differences, or motivated by interest group pressure. My goal is to bring all these perspectives together to paint as complete a picture as possible of what happened in these states. This is similar to what Jonathan Oberlander (2003) wrote about the politics of Medicare: "multiple theoretical lenses are necessary if Medicare's political picture is to be properly developed."

I build on the work done by many scholars using quantitative and qualitative methods to look at particular aspects of the ACA's implementation. These include a focus on partisanship and ideology (Burkey and Kamarck 2013, Jacobs and Callaghan 2013, Rigby and Haselswerdt 2013, Shor 2013), federalism and institutional fragmentation (Béland, Rocco, and Waddan 2014, 2016), and pressure from interest groups (Cauthon 2011b; Stiles 2013; Gray, Lowery, and Benz 2013; Callaghan and Jacobs 2016). Some have noted the important role of particular players, such as insurance commissioners (Haeder and Weimer 2013).

A number of scholars emphasize the benefits of thick description in policy analysis (Brown 2010). For example, Stonecash (1996) argues that the state politics literature needs to move toward a focus on explaining political processes and outcomes, and that the best way to do this is a methodological shift to comparative case study. McGrath (2009) warns, "measuring a process like implementation across states using a static set of criteria is not usually possible unless those criteria are so general as to be of only limited utility," and that a better approach is to examine factors affecting implementation within specific states.

The comparative case study method has a number of advantages over multivariate regression models for the questions I ask (Ragin 1987). First, inherent in this approach is a flexibility to use all pertinent data and to present it in a variety of ways, including qualitatively and quantitatively. Second, statistical power is significantly limited with only fifty cases. Instead, the comparative method accounts for every instance of a particular phenomenon. Even the most sophisticated quantitative methods to examine state decision-making obscure the nuances across time periods that are the very thing I am trying to explain.

I conducted more than two hundred semistructured interviews with leaders in twenty-four states between July 2011 and July 2016, including an average of eighteen people in the four case study states. These were the primary source of data for the case study chapters. Most interviews lasted 30–60 minutes and dealt with a variety of issues relevant to that person's role in the ACA's implementation. In each of the case study states I attempted to speak with an advisor to the governor, legislative leaders from each chamber, Republican and Democratic legislators on the relevant committees, legislative staff, bureaucrats in the state's department of insurance and department of health, and leaders of interest groups that lobbied on the exchange, including business groups, insurers, brokers and agents, hospital and provider associations, consumer advocates, and the Tea Party. I also spoke with leaders at the national level, including in the White House, the Department of Health and Human Services, and staffers to relevant congressional committees.

In exchange for their candor, I do not include any identity-revealing information without an interviewee's permission. Approximately 40% of the interviews took place over the phone. The rest were conducted in person, either in the participant's work environment or at a policy conference such as those run by AcademyHealth, the National Academy for State Health Policy (NASHP), the National Committee for Quality Assurance (NCQA), and the National Association of Insurance Commissioners (NAIC). I also approached these meetings as an ethnographer, taking extensive notes on the presentations, comments, and interactions among state and federal leaders. I went to Boise, Jackson, Lansing, and Santa Fe. I attended, watched, and/or read the minutes of every legislative hearing on an exchange in my four case study states, and took a similar ethnographic approach at these meetings.

I also rely on a variety of secondary sources such as government records and media coverage, as well as statistics and polling information from organizations such as the Commonwealth Fund, the Kaiser Family Foundation (KFF), and the National Conference of State Legislatures (NCSL). The State Refor(u)m document library developed by NASHP was helpful for obtaining copies of primary documents used by state policymakers and interest groups.[4] In one case I filed a freedom of information request under the Kansas Open Records Act to obtain a copy of a letter written by Governor Sam Brownback.

PLAN FOR THE BOOK

The next four chapters contain in-depth analysis of how Mississippi, Michigan, Idaho, and New Mexico made decisions about what type of health insurance exchange to establish. Each story is told chronologically so that readers experience the ups and downs of the debate as it unfolded. The chapters are organized into the same four time periods used by Jones, Bradley, and Oberlander (2014) to mark the phases of this debate: (1) March 2010–December 2010, when the ACA was passed to when outgoing governors and legislators were replaced in many states;

(2) January 2011–November 2011, covering the start of a new legislative session until when the US Supreme Court announced it would hear its first ACA case; (3) November 2011–June 2012, covering the 2012 legislative session and the Supreme Court's ruling; and (4) July 2012–October 2013, when President Obama was reelected and states made their final decisions leading up to the first open enrollment.

Chapters 2 and 3 focus on states that chose not to create an exchange: Mississippi and Michigan. In both cases the governor initially supported creating an exchange but faced strong resistance from the Tea Party. Governor Bryant of Mississippi ultimately opposed an exchange and successfully blocked an initiative led by the independently elected insurance commissioner, a fellow Republican. This made Mississippi the only state to have an exchange application rejected by the Obama administration. The Michigan story shows that even consistently strong support from a governor was not enough to ensure that a state would create an exchange.

I then turn in chapter 4 to Idaho, the only state in the country led entirely by a Republican governor and Republican legislature that chose to create an exchange. Like Mississippi and Michigan, there was strong Tea Party pressure to resist an exchange and a strong industry coalition in favor of local control. However, unlike the other two states, institutional conditions in Idaho allowed for pockets of expertise in the legislature. Under the leadership of Governor Butch Otter, these prominent legislators played a critical role in ushering health insurance exchange bills through the process. A new House Speaker and support from a group of fourteen freshmen legislators also proved pivotal.

Chapter 5 focuses on New Mexico, which also chose to create an exchange. The major differences here were that the legislature was controlled by Democrats and the Tea Party did not play a prominent role. As a result, the debate was less over whether the state should create an exchange—most were in favor—but the balance of power between the governor and the legislature in its creation and oversight. Governor Susana Martinez initially vetoed exchange legislation but then tried to set one up using an executive order. The legislature threatened to sue her for ignoring it, and the two branches eventually compromised at the last minute.

Finally, in chapter 6 I discuss the lessons from these four states, placing them in the context of how the rest of the country made decisions about health insurance exchanges. I highlight how the stakes of this battle were dramatically raised by the US Supreme Court's decision to consider the case *King v. Burwell*. I conclude by considering what this tells us about the ACA and the ongoing struggle for health reform, as well as the about the future of American federalism.

CHAPTER 2

Mississippi

INTRODUCTION

Mississippi is the only state in the country to have a proposal for an exchange rejected by the federal government. This was a fascinating outcome considering how badly the Obama administration wanted Republican-led states to run their own exchanges and given that former Republican Governor Haley Barbour had been trying to create an exchange in Mississippi for many years.

At first glance it may not seem surprising that Mississippi, a deeply red state, opted not to implement a major component of Obamacare. Barack Obama lost the state by 13 percentage points in 2008 and by 12 points in 2012 (Mississippi Secretary of State 2008, Mississippi Secretary of State 2012, see Table 2.1). Both US Senators have been Republican since 1989, and both voted against the ACA. In 2010, the four-person congressional delegation was split between Democrats and Republicans, although one Democrat joined the two Republicans to vote against the law. Republicans had won five of the previous six gubernatorial elections and in 2011 took full control of the legislature for the first time since the post–Civil War Reconstruction Era. The Tea Party and the very conservative wing of the party are largely credited with this takeover, which made it difficult for Governor Bryant and legislative leaders to support any component of the ACA.

Despite this partisan climate, two unique institutional features opened the door to the possibility of a state-based exchange. First, the Mississippi

Table 2.1. MISSISSIPPI'S POLITICAL AND DEMOGRAPHIC CONTEXT

Political Environment

- 2012 presidential election: Republican Mitt Romney (56%)
- Governor
  - 2003–2011: Haley Barbour (R)
  - 2012–present: Phil Bryant (R)
  - Term limits: two terms of four years each
- Mississippi House of Representatives
  - 2007–2011: Democrat majority, margin of 22
  - 2011–2013: Republican majority, margin of five
  - No term limits
- Mississippi Senate
  - 2007–2011: Democrats won a majority in the 2007 election, but enough Republicans switched parties by 2010 to give Republican a majority of two seats
  - 2011–present: Republican majority, margin of nine
  - No term limits

Demographic & Health Status

- Total population: 2,907,000
- Distribution of Population by Federal Poverty Level
  - Under 100%: 27%
  - 100%–138%: 9%
  - 139%–399%: 43%
  - 400%: 22%
- Distribution of Health Insurance Coverage
  - Employer: 45%
  - Other private: 4%
  - Medicaid: 20%
  - Medicare: 13%
  - Other public: 2%
  - Uninsured: 16%

Health Reform

- Joined lawsuit against the ACA
- Federal exchange
- Not expanding Medicaid

constitution in 1890 purposely created a weak governor out of fear that newly freed and enfranchised former slaves would elect one of their own to office (Shaffer and Krane 1992). The legislature was given strong oversight powers, and many executive branch officials are independently elected rather than appointed. Insurance commissioner Mike Chaney believed that as an elected official he did not need the governor's approval to lead the efforts of the Mississippi Insurance Department (MID) to create an exchange. Second, an earlier change to the statute governing the state's high risk pool gave Chaney broad authority over any state or federal insurance program in the state. He tried to use this authority to set up an exchange despite protests from Governor Phil Bryant.

The Mississippi story is largely one of conflict between two parts of the state's executive branch. The legislature was not a factor beyond mid-2011. At some points the major division was along party lines, though the major split was ultimately between Republicans. Interest groups also played an important role, with Tea Party and conservative leaders opposing an exchange while most stakeholders worked with Chaney's MID supporting its establishment (see Appendix A for a timeline of key events in Mississippi).

MARCH 2010—DECEMBER 2010

In the initial months after the passage of the Affordable Care Act, Mississippi's leaders debated whether the state would join the lawsuit and began exploring the extent to which they would participate in the law's implementation. Few major decisions were made during this period, though the continuation of previous debates and the shifting of political dynamics were extremely important for shaping the process going forward.

Haley Barbour Supports an Exchange

The debate in Mississippi over the creation of an insurance exchange predates the passage of the Affordable Care Act. Governor Haley Barbour's administration believed that the largest group of uninsured Mississippians was employees of small businesses (Interviews 2012–2014). As a result, he tried multiple times to create an exchange particularly focused on small businesses. In fact, a conservative pundit later wrote, "No Republican governor has been a greater fan of exchanges over the past few years than the most politically powerful of them all—Mississippi's Haley Barbour" (Donmenech 2011). Barbour explains that he learned of the idea from the Heritage Foundation and began working on it in 2007 after fellow Republican Mitt Romney created an exchange in Massachusetts (Interview January 2014). Ed Haislmaier and other leaders from the Heritage Foundation visited the state around this time and met with leaders to advocate for an exchange. Insurance agents and brokers opposed the concept because they felt it stepped on their toes, but a wide variety of stakeholders were open to the idea (Interviews 2013–2014).

Two bills creating an exchange were introduced in the Senate in 2008, one by Democrat Hob Bryan, and one by Republican Eugene Clark. The Republican bill to create an exchange as a not-for-profit corporation passed the Senate on a unanimous vote, though it was never brought up for a vote in the House. Democratic leadership in the House did not allow the bill to even come up for a hearing (MS SB 2833 2008). Governor Barbour pressed them to act in his 2009 state of the state speech before a joint session of the legislature:

> Last year I proposed the creation of a Mississippi Health Insurance Exchange to help small businesses and their employees get private health insurance. The Senate passed that bill fifty-two to nothing. The House did not consider it last year, and I hope you will join us this year in an effort to significantly increase the number of Mississippians with private health insurance (Barbour 2009).

A bill introduced in 2009 met the same fate, being passed with near unanimous support in the Republican-controlled Senate but never receiving a vote in the Democratic-controlled House (MS SB 2668 2009). Stakeholders do not remember the exchange being a controversial topic, but understood the position of the House leadership to be simple partisan politics: they opposed it because Republicans introduced it and Governor Barbour supported it (Interviews January 2014). A bill to create a legislative study committee to examine the issue passed both chambers the next year in April 2010, just weeks after President Obama had signed the ACA into law.

Governor Barbour's advocacy for an exchange did not mean that he supported the ACA. He argues that the version of an exchange he proposed was very different from an ACA exchange. "I got the bill introduced to create an exchange that was totally voluntary. No mandation at all. It was not subsidized. The purpose was to create a vehicle that the state, or a state-sponsored non-profit, could set up and manage, and that would create an administrative platform for small businesses to not only shop for insurance for their employees, but to get purchasing power to create a significant pool" (Interview January 2014). He strongly opposed the ACA (Shiner 2009) and pushed for the state to join the lawsuit against its constitutionality even though Democratic Attorney General Jim Hood refused. Hood was independently elected and felt he did not have to comply with the governor, to which a spokesperson for Governor Barbour responded, "The Attorney General is welcome to represent the people of Mississippi or the Governor will do that for him" (Hood 2010). Hood still refused, and Governor Barbour joined the suit on May 14.

Even as one arm of the Mississippi government was on the lawsuit to overturn the ACA, another was in the early stages of preparing to implement the law. On September 30, 2010, the MID received a planning grant from CMS of $1 million to conduct market analysis and develop a stakeholder engagement process to make decisions about what type of exchange would be created in Mississippi. The efforts were led by Insurance Commissioner Mike Chaney, though with general support from Governor Barbour, who saw this as an opportunity to use federal dollars to build the type of exchange he had been trying to create for three years. This might have set the stage for a conflict with the Obama administration over what qualifies as an ACA-compliant exchange. An aide to Governor Barbour described, "We're going to continue down the path of the exchange that we're doing right now because we've been doing it, and if the federal government has a problem with it, well, then they can come down here. And if at that point they don't feel like we need the grant money, then we'll cross that bridge when we get to it" (Interview March 2012).

Shifting Political Climate

Mississippi holds elections in the year before presidential elections, making it one of only thirteen states in the country to not hold gubernatorial and legislative elections in 2010 (NGA 2011). Even still, the rise of the Tea Party and the rightward shift in other states and in the congressional midterm elections had important implications for Mississippi politics, particularly in the state Senate. Although Democrats won a 28–24 majority in the previous election in 2007, by January 2011 enough Senators switched parties to give Republicans control of the chamber (Donatelli 2010). This change did not matter as much as it might have in other states, given the institutional design feature that it is the lieutenant governor that assigns committee chairmanships, not the senate pro tempore as in most other states. In other words, Republican Lieutenant Governor Phil Bryant already controlled the agenda even though Democrats held a majority of the Senate's seats after the 2007 election. In any case, the functional composition of the legislature did not change much, given that the legislators who switched parties tended to vote with Republicans even when they were Democrats. These shifts signaled the ascendency of Republicans in Jackson and the growing role of the Tea Party in state politics, foreshadowing the tension over implementing the ACA that would soon follow.

JANUARY 2011—NOVEMBER 2011

2011 marked an important turning point in the debate over whether or not to create an exchange in three ways. First, differing versions of authorizing legislation passed the House and Senate, though leaders from the two chambers failed to reach agreement and the bills died in a conference committee. This would be the last time the legislature would weigh in on the issue. Second, Insurance Commissioner Mike Chaney, with the support of Governor Barbour, decided to use the high risk pool as the vehicle through which to create an exchange. Third, the elections in November 2011 would determine who would be making decisions during the crucial implementation years of 2012 and 2013.

2011 Legislative Session

Four bills were introduced in the early days of the 2011 legislative session to create an exchange—three in the House and one in the Senate. One exchange bill emerged from each chamber in early February, with the House approving HB 1220 by a vote of 82–36 (MS HB 1220 2011) and the Senate passing SB 2992 44-7 (MS SB 2992). The Senate passed an amended version of HB 1220 one month later by a vote of 49–0, meaning versions of the same bill had passed both chambers and would become law if the chambers and Governor approved the compromise reached by a conference committee (MS HB 1220 2011). These votes reveal bipartisan support in 2011 for the concept of an exchange, with 91% of Democrats and 60% of Republicans voting for their chamber's version of HB 1220 (MS HB 1220 2011). These votes also reveal the extent to which exchange politics would shift in subsequent years. Some of the people who would later become the most vocal opponents of creating an exchange are on record voting for these bills. Senator Chris McDaniel, who in 2014 would emerge as a Tea Party challenger to US Senator Thad Cochran and would introduce bills to ban the state from creating an exchange, is the most notable example (MS SB 2464 2014).

Despite bipartisan support for the concept of an exchange passing in both the House and Senate, HB 1220 failed to make it out of conference committee and thus did not become law. The major differences between the two chambers dealt with governance. Democrats controlling the House preferred creating an exchange as a state agency, whereas Republicans controlling the Senate preferred that the exchange operate as a nonprofit entity disconnected from state government. Conference committee proceedings are not open to the public, and so it is difficult to know exactly what happened. A leader at the conservative think tank The Mississippi Center for Public Policy (MCPP) attributes the decision simply to "Mississippi's desire to uphold the U.S. Constitution" (Mississippi Center for Public Poilcy [MCPP] 2012). Informants explain that Republicans had greater leverage, given Governor Barbour's support for a nonprofit exchange, but Democrats were unwilling to compromise. Some speculate that Democrats were not entirely convinced that a loosely regulated exchange run by Republicans in Jackson would be better than a more tightly regulated exchange run by Democrats in DC, and so were willing to let these negotiations fail (Interviews 2012–2014).

Mississippi High Risk Pool

One reason Republicans were willing to let HB 1220 die without a compromise was because they believed they could create a nonprofit exchange within the state's high risk pool. This backup plan was possible because of an unrelated change to the risk pool statute in 2009 which gave the Mississippi Comprehensive Health Insurance Risk Pool Association (MCHIRPA) broad authority to help "citizens of the state who desire to obtain or continue health insurance coverage under any state or federal program designed to enable persons to obtain or maintain health insurance coverage" (MS SB 2842 2009). This language was added in response to the state's experience with the Trade Adjustment Assistance Reform Act (TAARA) Congress passed in 2002. The TAARA provided premium assistance to workers losing their job because their company went to another country. No insurers offered plans to this population in Mississippi, and when the high risk pool tried to step in, it was prevented by a restrictive statute limiting its activity beyond a narrow set of parameters. An official involved with the high risk pool explains that the broader authority added in 2009 was "so that if the state came along and asked us to do something else we wouldn't have to keep telling governors that we couldn't do it . . . This wasn't done with an exchange in mind. It was just simply to say that if the state wants something done, then this organization has the authority" (Interview January 2014).

Some people questioned whether the 2009 legislation really did give MCHIRPA the legislative authority to create the state's insurance exchange based on the 2009 legislation. There was talk of a lawsuit challenging this interpretation, though nothing materialized (Interviews 2012–2014). Governor Barbour was supportive of using the high risk pool, in part because it would ensure the exchange would be operated outside of government as a nonprofit entity. He turned exchange planning over to Insurance Commissioner Mike Chaney, who had rule-making authority and regulatory oversight over the risk pool. A conservative opponent of the exchange believes, "Some people later felt they had been duped and hadn't known they were opening the door to a state-based exchange" when they expanded the high risk pool's authority in 2009 (Interview January 2014).

The MID applied for a level 1 establishment grant within a month of being designated in charge of exchange planning. The Department of Health and Human Services (HHS) announced on August 12, 2011, that Mississippi would be awarded $20 million, making it among the first states to receive a level 1 grant. Accepting the grant opened the Barbour administration to criticism that it was taking Obamacare money at the same that it was challenging the law in court. An aide to Governor Barbour commented, "The Governor's perspective was that this is grant money, and the taxpayers of Mississippi have already paid for it through taxes, and we deserve our share of the pie. . . . We shouldn't reject [the grants] because of some ideology that's out there with some conservative Republicans, or conservatives, or think tanks, or whatever you want to say" (Interview March 2012). Republican US Senator Thad Cochran offered his support, saying, "I am proud of Governor Barbour's work to craft an insurance exchange program tailored to improve access to healthcare in our state" (Gillette 2011). Republican Insurance Commissioner Mike Chaney explained his view: "There are portions in that act that are good parts, and that happens to be the exchange. It's not a Republican idea. It's not a Democratic idea. It is a universal idea and it has been around a long time." While acknowledging the broader political dynamics, Chaney explained he had authority and autonomy that might not have been available to his counterparts in other states. "It appears that I am swimming upstream against the trend of other southern states, but here is the problem: other southern states did not have the statutory law that I had in place" (Chaney 2012).

How much flexibility would the Obama administration actually allow Mississippi in establishing its exchange? Unlike the exchanges described in the ACA, the bills Governor Barbour backed in 2008–2011 were focused only on small businesses and not the individual market, included no individual or employer mandates, and provided no subsidies to consumers. An aide to Governor Barbour anticipated conflict, explaining that the grant application submitted in the summer of 2011 was consistent with the type of exchange he had supported in the past. "You're never quite sure how it's going to fall out with HHS. But in his mind it was that we're going to continue down this path. The application that we turned in for the money, it was written like we were doing the exchange before—so we got the money based on the concept that we were touting all along. It's not like we changed what we were doing for HHS and then resubmitted the grant" (Interview March 2012). An official at the MID explained their strategy of being "super nice and cooperative now in the hopes that we might have more leverage later," but at the same time they would "do now, ask for forgiveness later" (Interview October 2012).

One of the first things the MID did with the money was go on an outreach tour to connect with stakeholders across the state and educate them on the exchange. An official in the department describes a week in the summer of 2011 in which they met with leaders in thirteen cities. "They were well attended generally. We got a lot of good feedback from people. People seemed to generally be in favor of the exchange concept. They were definitely in favor of the state operating it rather than the federal government" (Interview November 2011).

On October 18, Commissioner Chaney announced a formal process by which stakeholders would participate in developing the state's exchange. An advisory board consisting of eleven people would meet throughout 2012 to help make the major decisions. The board would include consumers, advocates, small businesses, relevant state government agencies, a federally recognized tribe, public health experts, providers, large employers, insurers, agents, and brokers. An MID press release explained that the number of seats on the board was expanded to thirteen due to "overwhelming positive response" (Mississippi Insurance Department 2012a). The first meeting was scheduled for January 2012, after the state's elections and after the start of the new legislative session.

2011 Elections

The 2011 gubernatorial and legislative elections were landmark events in Mississippi politics for two reasons. First, Haley Barbour was term-limited from running again and so a new governor was elected. As mentioned earlier, Mississippi's governor is comparatively weak, with limited formal powers to shape policy. Many people describe Haley Barbour as being more successful at using his informal powers of prestige, influence, connections, and money than any previous governor in Mississippi history (Interviews 2012–2014). He was previously a founding member of what has been described as the most powerful lobbying firm in Washington, DC, chairman of the Republican National Committee, and director of Ronald Reagan's White House Office of Political Affairs (Bipartisan Government Relations [BGR] 2012). Barbour's popularity and power solidified after his handling of the state's response to Hurricane Katrina in 2005 (Dao 2006).

Lieutenant Governor Phil Bryant won the 2011 Republican primary and general gubernatorial elections convincingly, but it remained an open question whether the increased clout of the governor's office would carry over or recede as Haley Barbour left office. Bryant's relationship with the Tea Party was an important new dynamic. The Mississippi Tea Party officially endorsed Bryant, with Chairman Roy Nicholson proclaiming, "We are granting Phil Bryant full right and title to claim to be America's first Tea Party governor!" (Hess 2011). However, the endorsement did not come until October 31, long after the more meaningful Republican primary, so it was unclear how beholden to this group Bryant would feel and whether the Tea Party would influence his stance on controversial policy issues such as an exchange.

Second, Republicans won control of both chambers of the legislature in November 2011, as well as every statewide office except attorney general. Republicans already controlled the Senate due to legislators switching parties in 2010, and this was the first time since Reconstruction that Republicans took control of the House. Insurance Commissioner Mike Chaney was also reelected, running unopposed in the Republican primary and winning 62% of the vote in the general election (MS Secretary of State 2011).

The results of these elections were important for shaping who would be making the major decisions on implementing the ACA over the next four years, though health reform actually played very little part in these elections. One reason is that Republican candidates for the key statewide offices, Phil Bryant and Mike Chaney, faced weak candidates. There was very little about Chaney's approach to the ACA for a Democrat to attack, since the state was one of the national leaders in working on an exchange. A former advisor to Haley Barbour also explained, "Democrats did not make a big deal out of [the ACA] because they're anti-abortion as well and didn't want to go down that road. Honestly, they couldn't have won an election if they had talked too much about it" (Interview March 2012).

Bryant regularly criticized Obamacare on the campaign trail, though he gave no indication that he opposed the exchange to the point that he would ultimately block the state's application. Many people remember Bryant saying he would allow the creation of an exchange begun under Haley Barbour to continue (Interviews 2012–2014). Haley Barbour points out that Bryant served in the powerful position of lieutenant governor and did nothing to stop each of the exchange bills advanced during Barbour's second term. "When I say the Senate passed my exchange legislation at least three consecutive years, that was with him presiding" (Interview January 2014). Even still, the people working on the creation of an exchange understood that elections have consequences. As one official described, "We have a whole other dynamic that is going to go into place in about a month. It's impossible to predict what's going to happen" (Interview November 2011).

NOVEMBER 2011—JUNE 2012

Writing about Mississippi's exchange debate in 2012, conservative state politics blogger B. Keith Plunkett argued, "it doesn't matter what positions Barbour had taken in the past, this is Bryant's baby now" (Plunkett 2012). With the expectation that Governor Bryant would either support his efforts or at least stay out of the way, Insurance Commissioner Mike Chaney continued the process of setting up the state's insurance exchange under the authority of the state's high risk pool. The exchange advisory board did the most important work during this period, giving interest groups an opportunity to shape the exchange's implementation and become invested in its development.

Exchange Advisory Board

The Insurance Department contracted with the consulting firm Leavitt Partners to facilitate the work of the exchange advisory board. The firm is led by Mike Leavitt, who was the governor of Utah before working as the secretary of the Department of Health and Human Services under George W. Bush. Some hoped that Leavitt's clout would legitimize an exchange for conservative opponents. Leavitt was part of the inner circle for Republican presidential nominee Mitt Romney and was tapped to lead the transition team should he win the presidency (Pear 2012). Leavitt's firm included people who had worked at the conservative organization The Heritage Foundation, which had supported the concept of an exchange many years earlier. The firm spent much of 2011 and early 2012 trying to convince state-level Republicans to move forward with an exchange. Leavitt explained, "I understand why some of my fellow conservatives oppose the formation of insurance exchanges, but continued inaction risks an Obama-style federal exchange being foisted upon a state" (Pear 2013).

Members of the insurance department's advisory board describe the process established by Leavitt Partners as orderly and transparent, allowing a wide variety of stakeholders to participate. The full board met monthly throughout 2012, with agenda items following a three-stage process. An issue would be introduced in the first month, presented more thoroughly in the second month, and decided in the third month. In the meantime, each of the ten subcommittees met to study the specific issues and make recommendations to the full board.

One board member says there was "much more consensus than I expected, largely because it was a good process." In particular, this person expected controversy around the determination of essential health benefits, with insurers pushing for bare-bones plans and providers and hospitals wanting everything covered. Instead, tension was minimal as all sides worked to find common ground (Interview January 2014). Another board member describes a similar experience and adds, "it wasn't for a lack of discussion. Everyone gave input, but it was measured. People wanted it to work and so they were trying to be reasonable" (Interview January 2014).

Not everyone involved was initially convinced that the state should run an exchange. Agents and brokers were among those who did not support an exchange but decided that if it was going to happen they wanted to be at the table shaping it. Each of the state's major insurers took the same approach, contributing to the exchange's development though remaining undecided on whether they would offer plans on the exchange. On the other side of the spectrum were consumer advocates who considered opposing a state-based exchange run by Mississippi's Republican leaders in favor of a stronger exchange run by the Obama administration. According to one advocate, they ultimately supported Chaney's efforts because "the Department of Insurance walked the talk" (Interview January 2014), and concluded state control would be better, even if run by conservatives. Stakeholders from a wide variety of perspectives say they felt heard and that the final decisions reflected the input they had given (Interviews January 2014).

Contracting with Leavitt's firm might have legitimized the exchange for some establishment Republicans opposed to the ACA, but not with the Tea Party. As one opponent described, "They could care less whether Leavitt was a Republican . . .. It does not play well that we are sending lots of money to some consultant in Utah to come set up our exchange here in Mississippi" (Interview January 2014). National conservative groups fed a suspicion for Leavitt Partners. Michael Cannon of the Cato Institute said, "It is strange to see Mr. Leavitt, a former Republican governor and former secretary of health and human services, helping and encouraging states to carry out this law for which Republicans have so much antipathy" (Pear 2012). Twila Brase of the Citizens' Council for Health Freedom, which worked to stop exchanges in other states, similarly stated, "Mike Leavitt is an enabler of Obamacare. He has taken advantage of Obamacare to expand his own business, instead of helping governors resist a federal takeover of health care" (Pear 2012).

However, the Tea Party in Mississippi had not played an important role in the debate to this point. An official at the insurance department explained in November 2011 that the Tea Party did not yet have much influence over policymaking in general in Mississippi (Interview November 2011). No one from the Tea Party attended the early advisory board meetings. At least if they did, they did not make their presence felt in any way. This would soon change in the wake of the Supreme Court ruling upholding the ACA as constitutional.

JULY 2012—OCTOBER 2013

There was uncertainty in June 2012 about what the upcoming Supreme Court ruling would mean for an exchange in Mississippi. The advisory board worked under the assumption that the law would survive and that they had tight deadlines to meet in order to submit a blueprint application in November. Some members wanted to continue building an exchange even if the law was struck down, though it is unclear that all stakeholders would have remained committed without the threat of a federal exchange. This high level of uncertainty was difficult for those involved, but was accepted as part of the process. As an official at the insurance department described, "We're used to adversity at this point. We've been doing this for a year and a half since the passage of the ACA. There's no use trying to predict tomorrow. We know today what the law is. If it's changed or our state takes a different approach, then we'll adapt accordingly" (Interview November 2011).

It was also unclear whether Barack Obama would be reelected that fall and what a Romney presidency could mean for the fate of the ACA, though none of this affected the expectation in Mississippi that November 16, 2012, was the deadline for the insurance department to submit an exchange blueprint application. The certainty that came with the Supreme Court's decision set in motion the three major events during this time period that would determine whether Mississippi would have a state-run exchange: (1) local Tea Party groups awoke to the issue and increased the intensity of their opposition, (2) the insurance department submitted its application for HHS's approval, and (3) Governor Bryant intervened and convinced HHS to reject the state's proposal.

Tea Party Mobilizes

The minutes of the July 11, 2012, meeting of the exchange advisory board include one sentence mentioning that Richard Wilbourn of the Mississippi Tea Party was allowed to speak. It says simply, "Mr. Wilbourn thanked Mr. Sisk (of the Mississippi Insurance Department) for allowing him the opportunity to address the Advisory Board, and proceeded to urge MID and the Advisory Board not to continue with establishing a state-based exchange" (Mississippi Insurance Department 2012b). Attendees of this meeting paint a much more dramatic picture of this event and describe it as an important turning point in Mississippi's exchange debate.

One board member describes noticing a particularly strong security presence in the lobby of the Woolfolk Building in downtown Jackson when he showed up for the July 11 meeting. He figured there must be a higher profile meeting happening that morning as well, but was surprised when he realized the crowd was there for the exchange meeting (Interview January 2014). Few members of the public had come to any of the previous meetings, but participants estimate that starting in July there were 20–30 people in attendance. The media must have been tipped off that they would be coming, because TV cameras were present for the first time.

The group of observers presented itself as the Mississippi Tea Party and insisted they be given an opportunity to speak. This is the first time anyone from the public had asked to participate and so the board had to develop a protocol for public comments. It decided that one person was allowed to speak per organization. Board members describe respectful conversations with the Tea Party members after the meeting. A board member who originally opposed the ACA told them he is sympathetic to their arguments, but feels they are going about this the wrong way. "They tried to sound smart but ended up looking bad." Another participant reflected, "They were nice folks and we tried to explain to them why we were doing this and that the consequence of their position would be greater federal control, but they didn't see that" (Interviews January 2014).

Although participants in the advisory board process describe a change in atmosphere once the Tea Party members started attending, there is no evidence this led to any substantive change in direction. The committees and subcommittees continued to meet, the website continued to be built, and the MID continued to prepare the state's blueprint application. The Tea Party did not weigh in on any of the specifics of an exchange and so did not influence the details of its development.

There is a bigger picture, however, with attendance at these meetings as one part of a broader series of developments by which the Tea Party gained momentum in mid-2012. The Supreme Court ruling was a galvanizing moment in which Tea Party members realized the ACA was likely to survive and they were running out of opportunities to block its implementation (Interviews January 2014). In addition to attending more advisory board meetings, a core group of Tea Party leaders living near Jackson met with Governor Bryant, encouraging him to oppose an exchange.

The MCPP—a state-level conservative think tank—played an important role in facilitating the growing Tea Party opposition. The MCPP wrote the reports and published the data that Tea Party members would use in their arguments. It also brought national leaders to Jackson to speak on why states should oppose an exchange, making a strong statement that this was the position conservatives should adopt. For example, Michael Cannon of the Cato Institute spoke at the MCPP Liberty Luncheon on July 12, 2012, the day after the Tea Party group first attended the exchange advisory board meeting (MississippiPolicy 2012a). The MCPP uploaded to youtube.com a brief encounter between Cannon and Insurance Commissioner Mike Chaney in which Cannon argued that the best way to flip votes in Congress to repeal Obamacare is for enough states to resist implementation. Chaney was put on the defensive, responding, "I came here today as a guest to listen to you, not to debate you. You have TV cameras rolling so you can get your point out . . . but unless Romney is elected, everything you have said is moot to a certain degree" (MississippiPolicy 2012b).

Another example of a national conservative leader visiting the state was Ed Haislmaier of the Heritage Foundation in January 2013, at the height of tension between Commissioner Chaney and Governor Bryant. In addition to testifying before a legislative panel on Medicaid expansion, Haiselmaier did radio and TV interviews and met personally with Governor Bryant. He acknowledged that Heritage supported the concept of an exchange years earlier, but argued that an Obamacare exchange is something entirely different. He further described that states will have to spend money on both the exchange and Medicaid expansion, but will get blamed when neither works (Interviews January 2014; Hess 2013).

By late 2012, the Mississippi Tea Party movement had created the same the conditions that allowed their counterparts to succeed in blocking exchanges in other states (such as Michigan), including a core of energized people committed to grassroots activism and a conservative organization supplying data and reports. The major difference in Mississippi was that the decisions were not being made by the legislature or the governor, but by an independently elected insurance commissioner and an advisory board of stakeholders supporting a state-based exchange. House Insurance Committee Chair Gary Chism speculated that the legislature could remove Chaney's authority to run an exchange through the high risk pool or could simply vote down a state-based exchange, though neither idea was seriously pursued (Hess 2013). Although the Tea Party was gaining momentum, it seemed to lack any levers of influence to stop the creation of an exchange. An opportunity soon developed.

At the July 11 advisory board meeting the Tea Party attended, Aaron Sisk of the MID mentioned that they were waiting to move forward on a couple issues until the Personnel Services Contract Review Board approved certain contracts with vendors (Mississippi Insurance Department 2012b). Perhaps this triggered the idea among Tea Party leaders in attendance to investigate how such contracts were approved and use this as a lever of obstruction. A recent report by the MCPP had already mentioned the Review Board as one of the administrative hurdles the MID had to pass over in order to hire consultants and information technology (IT) vendors to do the work of building an exchange (MCPP 2012). Preventing contracts from being approved would make it much more difficult for the MID to move forward.

The Personnel Services Contract Review Board is a relatively obscure panel of five people appointed by the governor. Its purpose is to "set forth rules and regulations, along with other pertinent information, that agencies should follow in the procurement of personnel services" for any contract in excess of $100,000 (Mississippi State Personnel Board 2012). The Review Board's website lists the dates and times of future meetings, but provides no information about upcoming agenda items (Mississippi State Personnel Board 2013). In other words, it is not easy for members of the public to know how to follow and attempt to influence Review Board decisions.

Jameson Taylor of the MCPP explains that the Tea Party started showing up at Review Board meetings and going through the exchange contracts under consideration around August 2012. As an example of what he describes as government overspending, Taylor recalls one contract charging the state $2,000 for rotating pictures in the website's banner, something he says that IT people tell him takes a half hour to complete and is virtually free (Interview January 2014). A member of the exchange advisory board's subcommittee that oversaw contracts describes the Tea Party presence at the state's Review Board meeting as unprecedented and notes that many of the contracts were held up as a result of this scrutiny (Interview January 2014). Another person describes, "Once they had been to a couple meetings and saw that contracts were delayed, that gave them impetus to go to more meetings and see what influence they could have" (Interview January 2014).

Even as they were succeeding in holding up contracts, the Tea Party felt that it did not have the power to ultimately stop the creation of an exchange. Mike Chaney had independent authority through the high risk pool and the White House was highlighting Mississippi's progress in national reports (White House 2012). At this point, the most some Tea Party members were hoping for was that the process would be more transparent (Interviews January 2014). However, many people on both sides of the debate believe that Governor Bryant took particular notice of the Tea Party's success in blocking the exchange's contracts. Bryant's opposition to Obamacare and the exchanges in general were known, but it was unclear how he would react to Mike Chaney's application to create an exchange. He ultimately decided to oppose Chaney, triggering an interbranch and intergovernmental feud lasting more than three months.

Bryant Opposes Exchange, Feds Reject Application

Despite the increased opposition, members of the exchange advisory board were pleased with their progress (Interviews 2013–2014). One person says they heard that only two or three other states were as far along. Another said, "We were basically ready, sitting on go. We had even already done lots of the testing and had really worked through lots of the details of the site" (Interviews January 2014). The site, www.onemisssissippi.com, went live in July, and an advertising campaign was under way by the fall. T-shirts were printed and an informational booth was set up at the state fair. Commercials featuring Mike Chaney ran on TV and on the jumbotrons at college football games in September.

Days after Barack Obama's reelection on November 6, Mike Chaney announced that the MID's exchange blueprint was ready to be submitted, but that he was waiting until he could present the details to Governor Bryant. Even so, he noted that as an independently elected commissioner of insurance, "I can submit the blueprint without the governor's approval" (Harrison 2012). Bryant did not respond, and Chaney's team grew frustrated.

The two men bumped into each other in a restroom on November 11 and Chaney confronted Bryant, asking why he had not returned his phone calls.

Bryant reportedly explained that he had been on a hunting trip out of cellphone range. In Chaney's words, "The governor asked me, 'What authority do you have to do this?' And I said, "Phil, what authority do you have to stop me?" (Epstein 2012). Bryant invited Chaney to meet the next day at the Governor's Mansion, where he explained that Republican governors have decided to unite in opposition to the exchanges "because [the Obama administration] will change the rules and control everything. You cannot trust them" (Epstein 2012). The Republican Governor's Association had just met in Las Vegas, with much of the meeting focused on opposing the implementation of Obamacare (Myers 2012). The nature of the issue had changed with increased pressure from the national party for state leaders to unify in opposition. Phil Bryant was among the Republican governors signing a letter calling on the Obama administration to extend deadlines and revise expectations (Vestal 2012).

Despite these conversations with Governor Bryant, Chaney submitted the MID's declaration letter even before Secretary Sebelius extended the November 16 deadline. He put out a statement asserting, "As an elected official and the chief officer of the Department of Insurance, I am authorized by state law to submit this Exchange Declaration Letter on behalf of the State of Mississippi" (Mississippi Insurance Department 2012c). Bryant immediately responded with a press release calling the exchange "a gateway to full implementation of ObamaCare in Mississippi," and saying, "This is one more step toward the largest entitlement program expansions in American history" (Bryant 2012a). This was Bryant's harshest statement against an exchange during the many years in which he was in a position to influence the debate. He was now in line with the state's Tea Party, who had recently vowed to make opposing "the Chaney/Obamacare Health Insurance Exchange" a top priority in 2013 (Pender 2012).

Bryant wrote Secretary Kathleen Sebelius eleven days later to formally register his opposition to Chaney's proposal, saying, "I feel compelled to notify you of my complete disagreement with this move. I am disappointed with the submission of that letter, and I am exploring my options" (Bryant 2012b). Chaney grew increasingly frustrated with the governor's opposition, particularly because he had been allowed to spend countless hours planning for an exchange without a hint that Bryant would oppose. Chaney wrote Bryant directly on January 4, saying, "Phil, there is simply no legitimate reason to impede the development of a state-based exchange at this point in time." Referencing Bryant's argument that the state will not actually have much control over the exchange, Chaney wrote, "I am confident that this is not the correct view to take on the subject" (Pettus 2013a).

The state's attorney general was consulted on whether Chaney had the ability to create an exchange without the governor's approval. Jim Hood issued a seven-page report on January 15 stating that the Insurance Department "is vested with authority to submit the application to establish a health insurance exchange," and, "Our office has found no statute which would allow the governor to override a decision of MID or the commissioner" (Pettus 2013a). Chaney celebrated this decision, saying, "We are very encouraged. Now everything will rest with HHS. The ball is in HHS' court." In response, Bryant's spokesperson dismissed the report as biased since Attorney General Hood is a Democrat and stated, "Governor Bryant will continue to resist efforts to further implement Obamacare, including a health insurance exchange" (AP 2013).

The decision was complicated by the federal requirement that each state's exchange declaration letter be signed by the governor. However, this was a rule promulgated by HHS and not in the ACA itself, so there was an expectation that HHS could work around a governor's opposition. The argument Chaney's lawyers made to HHS was that as an independently elected executive branch official, Chaney's signature actually satisfied this requirement (Interviews January 2014). One board member commented, "As far as the advisory board was concerned, they didn't need Bryant's signature. It wasn't through his office or the legislature, so he didn't need to sign" (Interview January 2014). Another board member remembers being concerned, but figured that the MID must have already worked all this out with HHS (Interview January 2014). According to one person working with Chaney's office, "We believe the governor doesn't get to tell the commissioner what to do. We think HHS agreed. There was ongoing dialogue throughout 2012 that led us to believe they would approve this. We also hoped the governor would come around" (Interview January 2014). The uncertainty over the disagreement with Governor Bryant was significant enough that the MID stopped its advertising and outreach activities in early January 2013 (MississippiPolicy 2013). Around this time, former Governor Haley Barbour called Commissioner Chaney to "just hang in there" in his efforts to establish a state-based exchange (Epstein 2012).

Jameson Taylor of the conservative MCPP observed that because Chaney is independently elected, Bryant's only two options at this point were to: (1) convince the legislature to change the high risk pool statute that Chaney was using to build an exchange, or (2) block an exchange by withholding Medicaid funds (Epstein 2012). The first option was unrealistic, given that the legislative session had just begun and that HHS's decision would be released shortly. Refusing to allow Medicaid to cooperate with the exchange seemed to be Bryant's only remaining path to stopping an exchange.

Three days after Attorney General Hood's report, Governor Bryant wrote another letter to Secretary Sebelius emphasizing, "In Mississippi, an attorney general's opinion is merely persuasive authority, not controlling law." Bryant went further in this letter than he had at any point to date. He argued that Chaney "lacks the necessary statutory and constitutional authority to establish and operate an exchange," and therefore HHS should consider any activity by the MID "null and void as a matter of state law." Acting on the idea Jameson Taylor articulated, he went on to write, "I am instructing the Mississippi Division of Medicaid not to assist or cooperate" with an exchange (Bryant 2013a). In other words, if HHS were to approve Chaney's application, Mississippi's exchange would be completely divorced from the state's Medicaid program. A lack of communication and coordination between the two programs would greatly complicate the establishment of a successful exchange. Members of the advisory board and others participating in the process describe being surprised by the governor's decision to use Medicaid this way, but still confident that their plans would move forward.

On February 7, HHS informed Chaney by phone that it was rejecting his exchange application. The letter from Gary Cohen of Centers for Medicare and Medicaid Services (CMS) that arrived the next day attributed this decision to "the Mississippi Governor's stated intent to oppose implementation of a state-based exchange." The letter also explained that a state-based exchange is required to develop and document a coordination strategy with other agencies' insurance affordability programs such as Medicaid. Cohen writes, "With a lack of support from your governor and no formal commitment to coordinate from other State agencies, we do not see a feasible pathway to conditionally approving a State-based exchange in Mississippi for 2014" (Cohen 2013).

Chaney held a press conference the afternoon he received the phone call in which he said he felt betrayed by the Obama administration. Describing the exchange planning process as "tap-dancing on a razor blade," he said "we've been working earnestly with these people for years, and we haven't waivered in anything that we've done." He went on to explain, "The decision came from the very top; it came from the White House. It wasn't HHS's decision, they were on our side. I think they were mortified." Reemphasizing the betrayal he felt, he added, "They've told the nation they want state-based exchanges, but here they are turning somebody down that's in the top three in terms of being prepared to operate an exchange." When asked why the White House turned down the application, Chaney speculated that they were afraid of a lawsuit challenging the MID's authority to operate the exchange and decided it would be better to implement a federal exchange than continue in the uncertainty that would result from ongoing litigation (MississippiPolicy 2013).

Governor Bryant released a statement later that day saying that HHS had not yet officially informed his office of its decision, adding, "I have said repeatedly that the health insurance exchanges mandated by ObamaCare are not free-market exchanges . . .. I firmly maintain my position that Mississippi will not willfully implement a mechanism that will compromise our state's financial stability" (Bryant 2013b). The governor released no other statement on this issue.

Tea Party leaders responded with appreciation for Governor Bryant. Members of the Mississippi Tea Party—along with Jameson Taylor of the Mississippi Center for Public Policy—met with Governor Bryant in the capitol building shortly thereafter and gave him a plaque honoring his "courageous and principled leadership in standing up for Mississippians constitutional rights" (TheMSTeaParty 2013). Janis Lane, president of the Central Mississippi Tea Party, put out a statement "applaud[ing] our Governor for his stand to protect the citizens and taxpayers of Mississippi against a federal government that is trying to usurp the rights of the citizens of this state." Lane's statement ironically attacked the Obama administration's reversal despite praising this decision, saying, "Kathleen Sebelius has revealed what many of us have known from the beginning—we cannot trust the federal government" (Mississippi PEP 2013).

Mike Chaney was publicly diplomatic in his statements about Governor Bryant's opposition. In the February 7 press conference he said, "Phil and I are friends. I hope this will not impair our ability to work together in the future. Reasonable people can disagree about an issue" (MississippiPolicy 2013). However, people who spoke privately with Chaney say, "he has a chip on his shoulder over this." One person said, "Chaney is pissed off at Bryant. He sees the Tea Party as largely responsible for railroading this process and no longer trusts Bryant" (Interviews January 2014).

Stakeholders involved in the debate over an exchange use words like "shocked," "disappointed," "sad," and "surprised" to describe the Obama administration's decision. One board member explained, "Through all this we really thought they would find a way. We had done a lot of work—A LOT of work—particularly in those final months. We had a very good blueprint that was certainly worthy of approval. Ultimately, I think HHS didn't want to get in the middle of a dispute between a governor and an insurance commissioner" (Interview January 2014). Even people who had been hoping for this outcome say they were surprised. One opponent of an exchange said, "I was shocked when the White House rejected our application. I would have assumed they would have approved the application and made the best of it and continue to pressure the governor to cooperate, and then fight Medicaid as a separate battle. I can't explain that. It was definitely a surprise" (Interview January 2014).

Many involved in the planning process believed the advisory board experience was productive even though the state did not end up operating its exchange. As one person described, "it had been beneficial to get all these people together" who normally do not communicate. But with no state-based exchange to operate, there was no reason to continue meeting. "It was like we all just shut down. No more emails, no more meetings. It just stopped. Many of the Insurance Department staff left shortly after, and so there was no continuity" (Interview January 2014).

Although the advisory board stopped meeting, the story of Mississippi's insurance exchange does not end in February 2013. The letter from CMS denying Chaney's application for a state-run exchange encouraged him to apply to do an exchange in partnership with the federal government (Mississippi Insurance Department 2013). Chaney opposed this idea, saying such an arrangement was "essentially the state doing the work, basically at our expense, to implement federal law. We're not going to do that" (MississippiPolicy 2013). The Obama administration provided a new possibility over the summer of 2013 in which the state could operate the small business SHOP exchange while allowing the federal government to operate the exchange for the individual market. Chaney took this option, using much of the work that had been done the year earlier as a foundation. There was little that Governor Bryant could do to stop Chaney because the SHOP exchange did not require any connection with Medicaid. "We clearly have authority to establish an exchange and operate a SHOP. I don't need his approval" (Millman 2013). Chaney submitted an application in August 2013, met with federal officials on September 18, and was approved on October 1 (Pettus 2013b). Ultimately, Mississippi has the type of exchange Haley Barbour had pushed for six years earlier. Barbour explains this outcome "suits me fine. Of the two, the small business exchange is far more important for Mississippi" (Interview January 2014).

The summer of 2013 was also dominated by political tension over whether the state should expand Medicaid. Mississippi policymakers describe their Medicaid program as one of the most micromanaged in the country, effectively needing to be reauthorized on an annual basis (Interviews 2013–2014). Complicating the dynamics is the fact that a supermajority of votes is needed each year, meaning that Republicans could not pass these bills on their own even though they controlled both chambers. Democrats attempted to force Republicans to consider the expansion, saying they would not support reauthorization unless an expansion bill was allowed to move forward. Republicans viewed this as a bluff and let Democrats protest. A special session was called in late June, with Democrats caving in the days before the July 1 deadline by which Medicaid would have expired. The existing program was allowed to continue for another year, but not without the ACA's expanded eligibility and federal funding (Whitaker 2013).

The interest group breakdown in the fight over Medicaid was similar to that of the exchange, with historically powerful groups such as insurers, hospitals, providers, businesses, and consumers mostly united in support of both an exchange and Medicaid expansion while the Tea Party and a handful of organizations opposed. In both debates, one of the major groups was seen as not playing as strong a role as many thought they should have, though it is unlikely that they could have changed the outcome. In both cases, the governor and legislative leadership ultimately sided with the Tea Party and opponents of implementing either component of Obamacare.

The outcome in Mississippi may have been different if Democrats had supported one of Haley Barbour's pre-ACA exchange bills, if the 2011 conference committee could have reached a compromise, if Governor Barbour had not been term-limited out of office, if Governor Bryant had not decided to block the MID, or if the Obama administration had decided to approve Mike Chaney's application despite Bryant's opposition. A state-based exchange would not have even been an option in Mississippi if the insurance commissioner was appointed by the governor, as in most other states, and if the legislature had not recently expanded the scope of the state's high risk pool.

An intergovernmental irony of the Mississippi case is that its exchange application was denied even though the state had taken the exact course of action federal carrots and sticks were designed to incentivize. Stakeholders responded to the threat of federal takeover and the promise of money and flexibility by developing their own exchange. However, Governor Bryant and the Tea Party did enough to block its creation, making Mississippi the only state to have an exchange blueprint application denied by the Obama administration. In this sense, it came closest to creating its own exchange without ultimately doing so. The fight over whether to create an exchange was largely decided through a fight over who gets to decide. This case exemplifies the challenge of giving states a prominent role in the implementation of federal law and serves as a powerful example of the ability of national, state, and local groups to use federalism and state politics to stand up to a national reform.

CHAPTER 3

Michigan

INTRODUCTION

Michigan appeared poised to be the first state led entirely by Republicans to create its own health insurance exchange as part of the Affordable Care Act (ACA). By November 2012, legislation to create an exchange had passed the Michigan Senate and was supported by Governor Snyder and the Speaker of the House. A broad coalition of interest groups lobbied in favor of a state-based exchange, including insurers, businesses, providers, hospitals, and consumer advocates. Even still, the House Health Policy Committee voted down authorizing legislation in November 2012, killing the possibility of a Michigan-run exchange.

The governor quickly shifted to pursuing a partnership exchange, receiving conditional approval for this approach from Secretary Sebelius in March 2013. Within weeks the legislature blocked the Snyder administration from spending federal grants, making it impossible to create a partnership exchange. Ironically, this time it was the House that sided with the governor and the Senate that stood in the way. Michigan had gone from nearly creating its own exchange to entirely defaulting to the federally facilitated exchange.

Michigan's role in national politics might have suggested a political environment open to implementing the ACA. Until Donald Trump, every Democratic nominee since Bill Clinton in 1992 has won Michigan, including Barack Obama with 57% of the vote in 2008. Since 2001, both of Michigan's US Senators have been Democrats. In 2012, President Obama and Senator Stabenow won reelection in Michigan with 54% and 59% of the vote (Michigan Department of State 2013), despite severe attacks from opponents about their roles in passing health reform (see Table 3.1).

Michigan's congressional delegation played a particularly prominent role in the national debate over health reform. Representative John Dingell (D) of Dearborn, who by the time he retired in January 2015 was the longest serving member in congressional history (Spangler 2013), introduced

Table 3.1. MICHIGAN'S POLITICAL AND DEMOGRAPHIC CONTEXT

Political Environment

- 2012 presidential election: Barack Obama (54%)
- Governor
  - 2003–2010: Jennifer Granholm (D)
  - 2011–present: Rick Snyder
  - Term limits: two terms of four years each
- Michigan House of Representatives
  - 2011–2012: Republican majority of sixteen
  - 2013–2015: Republican majority of eight
  - Term limits: three terms of two years each
- Michigan Senate
  - 2011–2012: Republican majority of twenty-four
  - 2013–2015: Republican majority of twenty-four
  - Term limits: two terms of four years each

Demographics & Health Status

- Total population: 9,714,000
- Distribution of Population by Federal Poverty Level
  - Under 100%: 19%
  - 100%–138%: 7%
  - 139%–399%: 40%
  - 400%: 34%
- Distribution of Health Insurance Coverage
  - Employer: 50%
  - Other private: 5%
  - Medicaid: 17%
  - Medicare: 15%
  - Uninsured: 12%

Health Reform

- Joined lawsuit against the ACA
- Federal exchange
- Expanding Medicaid

the National Health Insurance Act at the start of every session since 1957. He is also the author of the health reform bill that passed the US House in November 2009 (Dingell 2013). Representative Dingell was in the chair presiding over the passage of Medicare in 1965 and lent the gavel he used on that occasion to Speaker Nancy Pelosi (D-CA) to use when presiding over the passage of the ACA in March 2010 (Brusk 2010).

Similarly, Representative John Conyers (D) of Detroit has introduced the Expanded and Improved Medicare for All Act in every session since 2003, even after the ACA's passage (Conyers 2013). Representative Sander Levin (D) of Detroit was a prominent member of the House Ways and Means Committee during the congressional debate over the ACA, including serving as chair from March 2010 until Republicans took control of the House in 2011. Dingell, Conyers, and Levin were among the dozen or so people standing on the stage with President Obama at the bill-signing ceremony in the East Room of the White House on March 23, 2010.

Not all members of the Michigan congressional delegation were as pleased with the ACA as were Dingell, Conyers, and Levin, indicating that residents in parts of the state would likely not be supportive of its implementation. Bart Stupak famously led a group of antiabortion Democrats who refused to vote for the final bill until President Obama promised to sign an executive order upholding existing prohibitions on federal funding for abortion services. Dave Camp was the ranking Republican on the House Ways and Means Committee throughout the legislative debate over the ACA and took over as chair when Republicans won control of the House in 2011. He authored the Common Sense Healthcare Reform and Affordability Act, which he describes as "the only alternative [to the ACA] analyzed by the non-partisan Congressional Budget Office" (Camp 2013). Once the ACA passed, it was unclear how its opponents in Michigan would respond to the idea of creating a state-run insurance exchange.

Why did the state come so close to creating an exchange, only to default to the federal government? Four factors were particularly significant: (1) Governor Snyder's inability to convince enough Republican legislators to cooperate; (2) the surprising prominence of the Tea Party; (3) institutional design weakening legislative expertise, including term limits causing high levels of turnover; and (4) tension between federal and state timelines (see Appendix B for a timeline of key events in Michigan).

MARCH 2010—DECEMBER 2010

The reaction in Michigan to the passage of the Affordable Care Act was sharply divided. Within 10 minutes of President Obama's signing ceremony,

Michigan's attorney general Mike Cox (R) joined thirteen other states in a lawsuit challenging the constitutionality of the ACA's individual mandate and Medicaid expansion (Keyes 2010). Governor Jennifer Granholm (D) argued that Cox did not have the authority to join the lawsuit without her approval. There was little she could do to stop him, though she did take steps to lay the foundation for the ACA's implementation during the last few months before she was term-limited out of office.

Granholm Prepares for Implementation

Governor Granholm signed an executive order on March 31, 2010, creating The Health Insurance Reform Coordinating Council to oversee the ACA's implementation (Michigan Executive Order No. 2010-4). Speaking the next day at Sparrow Hospital in Lansing, she said that the reform would benefit Michigan, and that critics were spreading misinformation for political gain (Gaddis 2010). Janet Olszewski, the cabinet-level official in charge of the Michigan Department of Community Health (MDCH), was tasked with leading the council and facilitating coordination between state agencies. The agency received a $999,772 planning grant on September 30, 2010, which it used to solicit input from a variety of groups, including hospitals, providers, small businesses, insurers, unions, and consumer advocates. This was the first formal opportunity that Michigan's interest groups had to weigh in on what the reform would mean for Michigan.

Secretary Olszewski submitted the Council's report to Governor Granholm on December 2, 2010, recommending that administering its own exchange would put Michigan in a better position to coordinate eligibility with Medicaid and MIChild (the state's CHIP program). She argued that defaulting to a federal exchange would mean, "Michigan could lose control of its ability to determine its policy priorities." The desire for state control was strengthened by a lack of clarity over how a federal exchange would be structured. In the words of the report, "there is insufficient information to be able to describe how the federal government would operate an exchange for Michigan" (Olszewski 2010).

The Council recommended that a decision would need to be reached by February 2011 over whether the state would choose to operate its own exchange(s). Authorizing legislation should be passed by December 2011 with the financing structures developed by February 2013 if the exchange were to be online by October 2013. It also said that funds for exchange planning and implementation need to be appropriated each October between 2011 and 2013, and that by January 2015 the exchange must have a self-sustaining financing structure since no additional federal funds would be available from the federal government. As is shown throughout this chapter, the state fell well short of this timeline, ultimately rejecting control altogether.

Growth of the Tea Party

While Governor Granholm's administration laid the foundation for the ACA's implementation in Michigan, political battles over its existence continued in full force. Opposition to the law coincided with the growth of the Tea Party in Michigan. In the days immediately after Rick Santelli's "rant" on the floor of the Chicago Stock Exchange in February 2009, a small group of Michiganders used Twitter and Facebook to organize themselves and hold rallies across the state (Kremer 2009).

As health reform was making progress in Congress, Tea Party groups began transitioning their focus from the stimulus TARP bill to opposing what they labeled "Obamacare." Congress's inability to complete a health reform bill by the August 2009 recess meant that conservative activists had a month to mobilize constituents to vent their opposition personally to their legislators. Congressman John Dingell's town hall meeting in Romulus was a dramatic example of the growing level of animosity over health reform in the state. One intense confrontation happened when a father interrupted the meeting by pushing his wheelchair-bound son to the front of the room, pointing his finger at Rep. Dingell and yelling things like "your health care plan is going to take healthcare away from my son and kill him!" Anything Representative Dingell said in response was met with audience members yelling, "Liar!" This month of direct confrontation did not ultimately derail national attempts at reform, though it gave the growing Tea Party movement in Michigan an increased sense of purpose and confidence.

When the ACA was enacted the following March, Tea Party leaders began a petition drive to put the issue on the state's November 2010 ballot. A team of 300 volunteers collected approximately 150,000 signatures by July, falling 200,000 short of the state's requirement to put an initiative on the ballot. Jack McHugh, the senior legislative analyst at the Mackinac Center for Public Policy (pronounced Mack-in-awe), was part of this effort and responded, "Politicians who read this as public acceptance of the new law do so at their peril" (Gantert 2010).

Despite this failure, Tea Party groups formed the Mobile Action Patriot Strikeforce (MAPS) to try to influence the Republican primaries in August.

The MAPS built on "The Tea Party Activist Toolbox" published in 2009 by Jack McHugh of the Mackinac Center for Public Policy. The tool kit called for an aggressive style, saying, "Tea Party activists aren't impressed that their politician is a nice guy," and, "They're all nice guys, so get over it and ignore it. Hold them accountable for their deeds rather than their smile" (Braun and McHugh 2010).

This early involvement by the Mackinac Center shows that although the Tea Party was a grassroots movement in Michigan, conservative think tanks played an important role. They became a trusted source of information and inspiration.

2010 Elections

The 2010 elections half-way through President Obama's first term were more than a referendum on his agenda and accomplishments—they would determine who would be in power at the state level during the crucial ACA implementation years of 2011 and 2012. Among the candidates for governor was Attorney General Mike Cox, who accused fellow Republicans in the race of "failing to stand up against Obamacare" as he had done by signing the lawsuit (Cox 2010). Rick Snyder was arguably the least conservative Republican in the field, though benefited from the other candidates splitting the vote. Snyder emerged as an outsider, winning the primary and general elections.

Control over the Senate was never in question. Republicans held so many safe seats that they were unlikely to lose their majority, particularly in such a favorable election cycle. In fact, they strengthened control of the chamber, increasing their margin to twenty-four seats. The switch of party control in the House was dramatic and without recent precedent. Democrats went from a majority of 65 to 42 to being the minority by a margin of 47 to 63 (Michigan Department of State 2013). This gave Republicans their largest majority in the Michigan House since the early 1950s (Michigan Legislative Directory 2011).

This rightward shift in the legislature had enormous implications for the debate over health insurance exchanges during the next session, particularly in the context of term limits. Not only would both chambers be more conservative than in recent years, but a large percentage of members would be new to leadership or to the issue of health policy. The House Republican caucus chose thirty-nine-year-old Jase Bolger as the new speaker, making him the third straight person to begin their tenure as Michigan's Speaker with only two years of legislative experience (Christoff 2010). Of the top four Senate leaders, only one had previously served in the Senate and none had worked in health policy. The top four House leaders had an average of two years of legislative experience, with none having worked in health policy.

The membership of each chamber's health policy committees experienced nearly 100% turnover. The only exceptions were two Democrats who stayed on the House Health Policy Committee and Jim Marleau, who moved from being the minority vice-chair (i.e., ranking member of the minority party) on the House Health Policy Committee to chair of the Senate Health Policy Committee.

Stepping into this role at such an important time was a major challenge for new legislators. They lacked institutional knowledge of how to move legislation, substantive knowledge on the issues before them, and relationships to build consensus and compromise. Significant legislative turnover was also difficult for interest group leaders since the new people in charge were unknown quantities. An advisor to Governor Snyder explained, "before there were term limits, I would have known what the health chair was likely to do and what they are concerned about. Here I have no idea about any of those. It's a little bit foggier. And they probably don't either." This environment may have given interest groups greater leverage because "nobody knows enough to push back," (Interview June 2011).

As the new session was set to begin in January 2011, the foundation for political battles over an exchange was set. Opponents were gaining strength in their efforts to derail its progress in Michigan at the same time that Governor Granholm prepared the way for the incoming administration to continue with the ACA's implementation. Yet to this point, public discourse over the ACA was still focused on the mandate. Most policymakers were not talking about an exchange, and those who were would soon be out of power.

This transition period exemplifies the challenges of an intergovernmental approach to implementing federal law. The key players at the national level did not change, but the Obama administration would have to essentially begin from scratch with new state leaders. This episode also shows the limits of gubernatorial power. Any planning by the outgoing Granholm administration to this point could be undone or ignored by Governor Snyder and his team.

JANUARY 2011—OCTOBER 2011

Until January 2011, the debate in Michigan over the ACA and an exchange was largely theoretical, as the people who would be empowered to make key decisions had not yet assumed office. As the legislative session began, it was unclear which path Governor Snyder and legislative leaders would choose. By October, Governor Snyder had taken a strong stance in favor of creating a state-run exchange and enabling legislation he had helped craft was introduced in the Senate. The Governor took two particular steps to prepare the way for this bill: (1) holding stakeholder work groups throughout the first half of 2011, and (2) issuing a "special message" focused on health issues.

Stakeholder Work Groups

At his inauguration on January 1, 2011, Governor Rick Snyder told state leaders, "we have spent too much time fighting among ourselves and have become our own worst enemy" (Snyder 2011a). He spoke of expanding Michigan's economy and creating jobs, but did not once refer to the ACA or health reform. He was studying his options behind the scenes and developing a plan. Chris Priest, who had been the Director of Governor Granholm's DC office, was asked to stay and work in MDCH as one of the new administration's leaders on the ACA's implementation. Steven Hilfinger, director of the Department of Licensing and Regulatory Affairs (LARA) became another point person on the issue.

A Lansing-based consultant firm (Public Sector Consultants) was tasked with facilitating work groups to develop consensus about a health insurance exchange among a wide range of stakeholders. This was potentially redundant, given stakeholder input to the Granholm administration a year earlier, but an advisor to Governor Snyder described this as an opportunity for the new governor to take the temperature of key groups around the state. "It is always better to bring people in, interest groups, in from the beginning of the process rather than impose something on them, because no matter what you do they're not going to like it. The more buy-in you can get in the beginning of the process the better off you're going to be" (Interview June 2011).

A wide variety of organizations participated, including insurers, hospitals, consumer advocates, and academics. A final report was issued on June 17, 2011, detailing recommendations, with more than fifty receiving unanimous or "near-unanimous" support. The work groups recommended that Michigan develop its own exchange; that it should begin as an independent public authority (i.e., quasi-governmental organization) with the option of seeking nonprofit status at a later date; the exchange should be a clearinghouse instead of an active purchaser, meaning that it would not be the exclusive distributor in either the individual or group market; and the exchange should be funded through fees charged to carriers. A handful of participants opposed specific elements of these recommendations, though not a single person or group was opposed to Michigan taking control of its exchange (PSC 2011).

These recommendations were then presented to the legislature. The July meeting of the Senate Health Policy Committee was a particularly significant moment, as it was the first opportunity for groups to go on record either supporting or opposing the exchange. The work group report had not listed the positions organizations took on individual issues. The coalition of stakeholders testifying on behalf of the exchange was an unusual combination of groups typically aligned with Democrats such as the Michigan Consumers for Healthcare Advancement and the Michigan League for Human Services, alongside groups typically aligned with Republicans such as the Small Business Association of Michigan (SBAM) and the Michigan Chamber of Commerce (Michigan Senate Health Policy Committee, hereafter SHEAL, 2011). Supporting a state-based exchange was a bold step for many of these business organizations given that they had staunchly opposed the ACA during the 2009–2010 congressional debate. One business leader described support as a matter of pragmatism:

> I truly feel we have to be principled and we have to be pragmatic. Our job is to know which is which. Is this a stand on principle issue or this is not? Medicaid expansion and this are two examples of two very specific decisions that are before us. We weren't fighting about the whole law. We only had the decision about the type of exchange. Those who stood against it did so in a belief that they would be doing damage to Obamacare. We just didn't take that bet. We weren't willing to take that risk. (Interview April 2013)

Insurers also emphasized the role that states have traditionally played in regulating insurance markets:

> Once it became clear that this law would pass and things shifted to the state-level, we knew we wanted the state to run the exchange. We testified to that very early on. Each state is different. They have a different makeup. The population is different. Our insurance regulations are inherently different—most states are. We operate in a specific kind of way. Even though there were general guidelines that states would have to follow, we wanted as much control as possible to do it the way Michigan should be doing it. We were one of many groups who felt the same way. (Interview May 2013)

As important as this show of interest group support was, it was not clear which recommendations Governor Snyder would adopt and how the legislature would respond.

Snyder's Special Message

By June 2011, the Snyder administration decided to produce a "special message" on health and wellness. The message was released September 14, 2011, and included the governor's position on the health insurance exchange, as well as recommendations on how to address obesity, tobacco, food safety, and a wide variety of other public health issues. This would be the third such special message of his term, following one in March on local government reforms and one in April on education. Governor Milliken (1969–1983) used a similar approach as a way to set the legislative agenda for the following months. An advisor to Governor Snyder describes three components to these messages: "(1) what I'm going to do as governor, (2) what I'm asking the legislature to do, and (3) what I'm asking the people of Michigan to do" (Interview June 2011). A Democratic Senator said, "when they put a special message together, the full resources of the governor's office go behind those goals. They view these special messages as a checklist and focus on getting these things done" (Interview September 2011).

In his special message on health and welfare, Governor Snyder strongly advocated for a state-based exchange, saying, "I do not support a 'one size fits all' federal approach to health reform, which is where we would be if we were to allow the federal government to run a health insurance exchange." He went as far as saying that even if the ACA had not mandated the creation of an exchange, he would "still be in favor of utilizing technology to create a better customer service experience for Michiganders." In addition, Snyder advocated for the exchange to be established as a nonprofit entity, arguing, "the legislature should not create a duplicative regulatory structure for health insurance in Michigan" and "should encourage healthy competition rather than simply add new transaction costs to the expenses that individuals and small businesses already face." He further added that the exchange should not be the only available option for customers to purchase insurance (Snyder 2011b).

The debate over the content of the health and wellness special message took place mostly behind closed doors, with significant input from committee leaders from each chamber. An advisor to Governor Snyder described this process as trying to facilitate many of the big compromises before legislation is even introduced. "The more you can work out up front, the better off you'll be when you engage in the legislative process. That's what we're trying to do" (Interview June 2011).

Participants of the work group process later expressed frustration over not knowing how their recommendations were incorporated, particularly given that Snyder called for the exchange to be a nonprofit entity after they had recommended it be a quasi-governmental organization (Interviews 2011–2013). Those involved in crafting the special message say that the work group recommendations were given serious weight, but that the governor knew from the beginning that he wanted a nonprofit exchange. As one legislative staffer put it, "A quasi-governmental organization wasn't really discussed too closely. The goal is to remove it further from government" (Interview September 2011).

Chris Priest noted, "Governor Snyder's focus is on being consumer friendly and valuing customer service. We felt that [a nonprofit entity] would be the best way to do this. We wanted to set up a structure that would be flexible and as much outside of government as possible, something that would be forced naturally to keep its costs low" (Interview May 2013). There was also a political motivation to this approach, with the expectation being that a clearinghouse exchange run as a nonprofit housed outside of government would be the most likely to win support from Republicans in the legislature.

Not only were the proposals tailored to appeal to the right, but so were the words to describe and sell the proposals. Careful attention was paid to frame an exchange to appeal directly to conservatives by emphasizing markets and competition. In the weeks leading up to its release, a Republican legislative staffer said they would be surprised if the message even used the phrases "Affordable Care Act" or "insurance exchange" (Interview September 2011). Instead, the governor called his proposed exchange "The MI Health Marketplace," (pronounced My Health Marketplace). The federal government soon adopted this nomenclature, insisting that the word "exchange" be replaced with "marketplace."

The roll out of the message was designed to give momentum to the governor's proposals. A press conference was held at the Heart of the City Health Center in Grand Rapids.[1] These events were coordinated with legislative leaders so that the next day, Steven Hilfinger and Shelly Edgerton from LARA and Chris Priest from MDCH testified on the MI Health Marketplace before a special joint session of the Senate Health Policy and Insurance Committees. They were immediately followed by Olga Dazzo, director of MDCH, and two of her deputies presenting on other elements of the special message (Michigan House Health Policy Committee [MI HHEAL]

2011). Similar presentations were subsequently made in the House (MI HHEAL 2011a, 2011b).

The timing of the special message coincided with efforts by the Snyder administration to apply for a federal level 1 establishment grant. The state asked for nearly $10 million from the federal government to conduct studies and plan for the creation of an exchange. The receipt of this grant would ultimately be controversial with the legislature, but it was not when the application was submitted in the fall of 2011.

Snyder's special message held to the timeline recommended by the Granholm administration, challenging the legislature to have a bill on his desk by Thanksgiving. Both chambers of the legislature initially seemed supportive. A key staff person for the House Health Policy Committee (the committee that ultimately defeated the legislation) commented, "Our goal is to have our legislation on the governor's desk by Thanksgiving. That is the Senate's goal as well. That gives us two, two and a half months. That is our goal. We do want to meet the deadlines for meeting the qualifications and criteria to receive grants. We would like to receive all the federal money we can" (Interview September 2011). A member of the Senate Health Policy Committee said they would be surprised if legislation creating a state-based exchange was not enacted by the end 2011 (Interview September 2011).

The special message's roll-out was not entirely smooth, though not because of the governor's position on health insurance exchanges. In fact, the most controversial elements of the message had little to with the ACA. The media focused most of its attention on proposed requirements to mandate insurance coverage for treatments related to autism in children and for each child's body mass index (BMI) to be reported to the state annually (Thoms 2011). The Chamber of Commerce quickly linked these proposals with the ACA, saying, "Across the state, employers and individuals were angry at the passage of Obamacare and its focus on more governmental control and top-down mandates. Make no mistake: Support for more health care mandates is tantamount to adopting the same government control and cost-shifting at the heart of Obamacare" (Michigan Chamber of Commerce 2011).

Although not directly related to an exchange, this was an inauspicious beginning to the debate that was about to take place in the legislature over MI Health Marketplace. The Chamber of Commerce and other business groups advocated on behalf of a state-based exchange, but this message was often confused or drowned out by their strong opposition to the ACA as a whole and to Snyder's other health policy proposals.

Opposition Continues to Grow

Opposition to the ACA continued to grow as Governor Snyder advanced plans to create an exchange. Animosity came most strongly from three sources: (1) national organizations, (2) state-level organizations such as the Mackinac Center for Public Policy and the Michigan chapter of Right to Life, and (3) grassroots organizations. First, Governor Snyder resisted pressure from national groups such as Cato, ALEC, and the Republican Governors Association to return money or otherwise resist implementation. Most notably, he was the only Republican governor not to sign a letter calling for the ACA's repeal and greater flexibility on Medicaid (Republican Governors Association [RGA] 2011). Advisers to Governor Snyder described the decision to not return grant money and not sign the letter by saying, "It's a simple decision. That's the way the governor looked at it. We're not going to get in a state's rights debate. There is no sense in doing that stuff. First, the odds of this being entirely repealed are slim to none, so you do a reality check. Second, it is federal law. Third, he's more interested in Michigan than he is in the national debates" (Interviews 2011–2013).

Opposition at the state level was largely driven by the Mackinac Center for Public Policy. Based in Midland, the Mackinac Center has been called the "the largest right-wing state-level policy think tank in the nation" (Steimel 2013). The Center is part of a broader organization called the State Policy Network, which describes itself as "made up of free-market think tanks fighting to limit government and advance market-friendly public policy at the state and local levels" (SPN 2013). Mackinac's leaders have trained many of the people running sister organizations around the country and have participated in ALEC task forces focused on health reform (Sourcewatch 2013).

The Center takes a multipronged approach to attempting to influence public policy in Lansing. In addition to issuing reports based on independent research, it publishes blog posts, runs a news service called Michigan Capitol Confidential (CAPCON), and has a legislative tracking service called Michiganvotes.org. During the summer and early fall of 2011, Mackinac used each of these outlets to publish arguments against the creation of an insurance exchange. Senior legislative analyst Jack McHugh wrote most of these pieces, in many cases disseminating information from national organizations such as Cato. In these reports, McHugh argued that creating an exchange would "lend the appearance of legitimacy to the law," thus undermining the judicial challenge (McHugh 2011a). He also argued, "there is no such thing as a state-run exchange," since everything needs to be approved by the federal government and because interest groups would have too great an influence (McHugh 2011b, 2011c). These articles published by the Mackinac Center became the basis of the arguments used by the Tea Party and opponents of an insurance exchange.

At the same time that a major piece of his agenda was being challenged from the right, the governor was facing a recall challenge from the left. The Committee to Recall Rick Snyder worked throughout the summer of 2011 to try and collect the 800,000 signatures needed to put a recall of Governor Snyder before voters (United Press International [UPI] 2011). Much of this group's anger was directed at a law signed by Governor Snyder in March that gave broad powers to emergency financial managers appointed by the state, including the ability to supersede elected officials and terminate union contracts. An estimated three thousand people filled the Capitol Building protesting the law the day Snyder signed the bill into law (Mudgett 2011). The issue attracted national attention, with Jesse Jackson visiting the state calling for civil disobedience (Bien 2011) and Rachel Maddow criticizing the law on her MSNBC show (Maddow 2011). The campaign to recall Rick Snyder ultimately fell short, collecting 500,000 by the deadline at the end of September 2011 (Bowers 2011), although enough signatures were ultimately collected to put a referendum of the new emergency manager law on the November 2012 ballot (Hoffman 2012).

It was against this backdrop of a divided right and an angry left that legislation to create MI Health Marketplace was introduced in the Senate on September 22, 2011, by Senator Jim Marleau of Oakland County.

NOVEMBER 2011—JUNE 2012

November 2011 was an important turning point in the debate over whether to create an insurance exchange. The bill SB 693 to create MI Health Marketplace passed the Senate on November 10. Days later on November 14, the US Supreme Court announced it would hear the cases challenging the constitutionality of the ACA. This cast a shadow over deliberations in the Michigan House that was difficult for supporters to overcome. A Republican House staff member would later admit that regardless of the public comments about passing a bill by Thanksgiving, they never intended to bring the bill up for a vote once it became clear the Supreme Court would hear the ACA's case (Interview February 2012).

SB 693 in the Senate

Jim Marleau, chair of the Senate Health Policy Committee, took the lead in pushing SB 693 through the Senate. Supporters had three advantages in their favor as the bill made its way from the Senate Health Policy Committee to the Senate floor. First, they had the support of Governor Snyder, who had come out strongly in favor of a state-based exchange and had devoted his administration's resources at LARA and MDCH to planning activities. It was not immediately apparent that his support would be an asset. Legislative staff members in both chambers describe a strained relationship with the governor during the early months of his administration, in part due to his campaign promise to change the way business is conducted in Lansing. As one Republican Senate staff member described, there was "an expectation that once he arrived they would teach him what is going on and how things really work. He would be put in his place and it would be an adversarial relationship" (Interview September 2011). Instead, this person described Snyder as "an out of the box thinker who is pro-active in working with legislators and in seeking them out. It hasn't been adversarial. I have become a fan."

A staff member to a House Republican in leadership echoed these sentiments about the governor's relationship with legislators in early 2011, particularly as Snyder took a strong stand on the exchange. "Keep in mind that the Republican that was elected governor was not the establishment candidate everyone thought was going to win. He was not active in Republican politics; he had a business background. This attracted Michigan voters. Now he is in office and to his credit looks at issues not first from a political bent, but from a CEO perspective. When he looked at the exchange, he thought it made sense." This person went on to add, "most Republicans in the House and Senate thought he lost his marbles" by supporting an exchange. "Does he understand politics? This is perhaps a cornerstone issue in the upcoming election and at the very least we should wait to see how this plays out. To his credit, he didn't wait" (Interview May 2013).

Instead, the Snyder administration engaged in an aggressive legislative strategy. Chris Priest and Steven Hilfinger took the lead in testifying before multiple committee hearings, holding numerous meetings with groups of legislators and their staff, and meeting one on one with each senator on the Health Policy Committee, as well as others in the Republican and Democratic caucuses. The dynamic between branches of government was complicated by the fact that the legislature had already taken a number of tough votes by this point in the session, including the emergency manager bill and a proposal that paid for the elimination of a business tax in part by increasing personal income taxes on pensions and other retirement income (Luke 2011). He was also trying to enact education reforms and win approval for a new bridge between Detroit and Canada.

The second potential advantage for supporters of an exchange was the broad set of interest groups in their corner. This was not a coalition in the sense that groups coordinated every activity, though their efforts were complementary. The Small Business Association of Michigan (SBAM), which some have called one of the most influential groups in Lansing (Interviews 2013), aggressively worked the phones and attended meetings with legislators. Other groups such as Blue Cross Blue Shield of Michigan were similarly engaged in lobbying senators. Trinity Health, the hospital chain headquartered in Livonia, Michigan, brought in experts such as Jon Kingsdale—who led the creation of the Massachusetts exchange in 2006—to speak to legislators and lobbyists about the path ahead.

The third advantage was that Senators would not be up for reelection again until 2014. Unlike states like Idaho, where all senators are up for reelection every two years, and Texas, where senators serve four years but elections are staggered so that half the body is on the ballot every two years, all of Michigan's thirty-eight Senators serve four year terms on the same electoral cycle. Legislative insiders feel that this gave senators a little more room in 2011 to examine the policy merits of SB 693 compared to the House, where members are on the ballot every two years (Interviews 2011–2013).

Senator Marleau spoke to the Republican caucus about the exchange in early September 2011, trying to convince them this is not the equivalent of implementing Obamacare in Michigan. He did not bring up access, rather trying to sell it as a way to control costs. Marleau was quoted as saying something along the lines of, "This is not Obama-style reform. This is a Republican idea. This is the Michigan solution" (Interview September 2011). Interest group leaders were frustrated that despite all the policy reasons they felt Michigan should run its own exchange, they "had to frame it as being about state's rights. You had to find a way for people to support this without saying they support Obamacare" (Interview May 2013).

At the same time, supporters faced the challenge of finding a way to convince enough Republicans to sign on without alienating too many Democrats and liberal groups. Michigan legislators joke about there being a special Lansing zip code of 56-20-1, since this is the number of votes needed to pass legislation through the House and Senate, and to be signed by the governor. Republicans held enough seats in both chambers that they could pass legislation without needing a single Democratic vote. However, given the divisions among Republicans, the most likely path in each chamber would be to secure support from as many Democrats as possible and then as many Republicans as necessary to make up the difference. In 2011 there were forty-six Democrats in the House, meaning that if they all supported an exchange, only ten House Republicans would need to vote in favor. The calculus was similar in the Senate, with only eight Republicans needed to join the twelve Democrats.

An advisor to Governor Snyder expected legislators "to be all over the map in terms of how they react to an exchange. Most Republicans are saying we should do it like Utah. Most Democrats are saying we should do it like Massachusetts. We're trying to find the middle ground—the Michigan way. At the end of the day all that matters is 56-20-1. Our job is to get the 56, 20, and 1. Well, to get the 56 and 20—we have the 1!" (Interview June 2011). Senate Democrats supported an exchange, though there were some feelings of discontent under the surface. As the leader of a liberal organization described, many supported SB 693 even though they felt it did not go far enough. They hoped the Michigan exchange "would evolve from a clearinghouse exchange to an active purchaser where the choices are a little more selective. . . . The Marleau bill wasn't perfect, but it was reasonable. We could have worked with it and improved it over time" (Interview May 2013).

After clearing the Senate Health Policy Committee, SB 693 was approved on the floor by a vote of 25–12 on November 10, 2011. All twelve Democrats voted in favor and were joined by thirteen Republicans, exactly half the Senate Republican caucus (Michigan Senate Roll Call #663 2011). It was not an easy vote for Republicans, with Senators such as Rick Jones of Grand Ledge saying he had to "hold his nose" while voting for the bill (Associated Press [AP] 2011b). Senator Patrick Colbeck (R) of Canton used a floor speech to remove his name as a cosponsor of the bill. He said:

> I rise in strong opposition to SB 693. My original co-sponsorship commitment was predicated on the understanding that this bill would provide a free market alternative to the Federal "Affordable Care Act." As a co-sponsor, I had worked hard to ensure that the bill would live up to this promise. My concerns have not been addressed in this version of the bill and I have read it thoroughly. Rather than serving as a free market alternative, I have come to the conclusion that this bill would simply further enable the implementation of the Affordable Care Act, commonly known as Obama-care. (Colbeck 2011)

Senator Colbeck asked for time to submit "a vetted alternative" that would narrow the scope of the MI Health Marketplace from performing "all exchange duties" to focus on determining eligibility for government assistance to citizens" (Colbeck 2011). His name was removed from the bill, but the vote carried on.

The Tea Party was paying attention to the Senate's bill but did not fully mobilize. On her blog the next day, Tea Party activist Joan Fabiano said this was because the Senate pushed the bill through without normal debate. Fabiano was one of the original leaders of the Tea Party movement in Michigan and was connected online to other activists. They reacted strongly to the bill's passage, issuing a call to arms for the Tea Party to act aggressively as SB 693 moved to the House. Republicans who supported the bill were accused of "putting their career over principles" (Fabiano 2011a). A political action committee run by the RetakeOurGov Tea Party Group used the moment as a fund-raising tool, telling supporters, "The passage of SB 693 was a deliberate poke in the eye to the Tea Party. We cannot just ignore this direct assault on our values. We have worked too hard and too long to fight Obama Care to give up now" (Retakeourgov 2011).

Negative attention from the Tea Party was uncomfortable for Republican Senators. Senator Judy Emmons tried to deflect criticism for voting for SB 693 by introducing a resolution on the same day "to express support for the continued efforts of the Michigan Attorney General to oppose the implementation of Obama Care and to memorialize Congress to repeal it" (Michigan Senate Resolution [SR] 95 2011). The resolution narrowly passed 20–17 with support from all thirteen Republicans who also voted for SB 693 (Michigan Senate Roll Call #664). The resolution did little to appease activists, who called it a "duplicitous move" and wrote, "Did they really think we should be fooled by this? What an insult to the people of Michigan!" Fabiano predicted the House would act quickly, and she and others vowed that the Tea Party would be ready (Fabiano 2011a).[2]

With the Senate having moved quickly to pass SB 693, the bill's fate was largely in the hands of Speaker Jase Bolger and Representative Gail Haines, chair of the House Health Policy Committee Meeting.

SB 693 Stalls in the House

As the debate shifted from the Senate to the House in mid-November 2011, it was clear that SB 693 would not meet Governor Snyder's timeline of being enacted by Thanksgiving. Having a bill passed by the time the legislative session closed at the end of the calendar year became the new goal for supporters of an exchange (Interviews 2011–2013). This was not as hard a deadline in Michigan as it would be in other states. When the 2011 legislative session ended in Idaho and New Mexico for example, all legislation that had not passed was dead and would have to begin the process again. Bills in Michigan operate on a two-year cycle, so that SB 693 was still viable legislation until December 2012.

When the House reconvened in January, the House Health Policy Committee continued studying its options. Between September 8, 2011, and January 19, 2012, the House Health Policy Committee held ten hearings on the exchanges, including every Thursday morning between October 6 and November 10. One senior staff member said in their fifteen years in Lansing they had not seen more committee deliberations on an issue than were held about the exchange (Interview May 2013). Each meeting included testimony in support of an exchange by representatives of state agencies, practitioners, insurers, businesses, and consultants working in other states. The meetings also provided an opportunity for citizens to offer brief testimony or file a written statement indicating their support or opposition of an exchange. Despite having so many hearings, no vote was held during this period.

Republican leaders had both policy and political reasons for delaying a vote in the House. First, they felt that with so many unknowns about the fate of the law it would not be prudent to proceed with the creation of a state-based exchange. The Department of Health and Human Serices (HHS) had not yet released final regulations on an exchange, and policymakers were frustrated about a lack of clarity over their options and requirements. How could they choose whether they preferred a state or federally run exchange if they did not know details about the federal model? Similarly, they worried that once HHS's final regulations were released, the state would be stuck with hidden costs or would have to spend resources revising elements of its exchange. The safer thing, they felt, was to wait and let the judicial process play out.

Richard Murdock, executive director of the Michigan Association of Health Plans made the case that delaying would be a self-fulfilling prophecy for opponents, leaving the state too little time to establish an exchange after the Supreme Court ruling (Murdock 2012). A spokesperson for House Speaker Bolger responded, "there's plenty of time to get something in place" after the Court rules, adding, "If people are dedicated, this can get done" (Associated Press 2011c). The director of LARA, Steve Hilfinger, responded, "If we wait until June to move forward on that, the odds of us being able to satisfy HHS that we have an exchange in place . . . would be nonexistent. We certainly don't want to lose six months of planning time and seal our fate with a federal exchange. That would be devastating for Michigan" (Associated Press 2011c).

Michigan was one of the few states that had the option of delaying its decision with the realistic possibility of still taking a vote in 2012. Only nine states had sessions running into July, and the Supreme Court's ruling was expected at the end of June, meaning that very few other states could wait for the ruling and still pass legislation creating an exchange—at least without calling a special session, an unlikely prospect so close to the election (Jones 2012). Ironically, the ability in Michigan to make decisions later gave opponents an excuse to stall. Without the tight deadline of a session end date, opponents felt little pressure to rush. Even so, the final deadline for a level 2 establishment grant—the major source of funding for beginning a state-run exchange—was June 29, almost immediately after the end of the Supreme Court's session.

One interest group leader called this period "the triple dog dare" phase of the exchange debate because Republican lawmakers felt HHS was bluffing on its threats. Another interest group leader quoted Chairwoman Haines saying HHS would never actually come in and set up an exchange (Interview April 2013). A House Republican staff member said that the Obama administration wanted red states to do an exchange so badly that they would eventually cave on deadlines and would "let us do whatever we want" (Interview February 2012). A Tea Party leader said HHS "couldn't and they wouldn't" run exchanges for all the states that chose not to do one on their own (Interview May 2013). Opponents admitted that they had little to lose by stalling, since they did not believe they would gain much control if they did an exchange anyway (Interviews 2011–2013).

House Republican leaders felt that creating an exchange brought little political benefit but potentially significant risk: 2012 was an election year for every member of the House, with the filing deadline for the primaries right around the corner in May. Groups such as the Tea Party and Americans for Prosperity were becoming increasingly vocal and aggressive on this issue. A Republican senior staff member said they had verbal support from enough people that they were confident SB 693 would pass if it reached the floor (Interview December 2011). However, many Republicans were nervous about the tough votes they had already taken and did not want to take a risky vote on Obamacare if they did not need to. After the December 1 meeting of the House Health Policy Committee, House Republican leaders announced that no vote would be held until after the Supreme Court's ruling (Interviews 2012–2013).

House Blocks Federal Grant

As it turned out, there was an important Obamacare vote much sooner, though not on the creation of an exchange itself. The federal government awarded the state a $9.8 million level 1 establishment grant on November 29. LARA had applied for this grant two months earlier "to conduct additional analysis on the impacts of the Exchange and the Affordable Care Act in Michigan," including market analysis, technology planning, and education and outreach (Centers for Medicare and Medicaid Services [CMS] 2014). This grant was seen as a natural progression from the $1 million planning grant received a year earlier and was not expected to be controversial. Policymakers on both sides of the aisle were asking for more detailed information than the state had available, and the Snyder administration said they wanted to use the grant to develop answers to these questions.

Accepting this grant did not commit the state to create an exchange, though conservative leaders such as Jack McHugh at the Mackinac Center warned, "state cooperation and grant-seeking may further entrench Obamacare, making it harder to eventually invalidate or repeal" (McHugh 2011d). Joan Fabiano similarly called for the state to reject this grant (Fabiano 2011b). Governor Snyder made it clear he would not follow the lead of other Republican governors who rejected their federal grants (Interviews 2012–2013). However, the Michigan Constitution also requires the legislature to approve any executive spending, even of money received by federal grant.

On the same day in November 2011 that the Senate passed SB 693 to create an exchange and Resolution 95 to express support of Michigan's participation in the lawsuit, the Senate also passed a $366 million supplemental appropriations bill by a vote of 28–8, authorizing LARA to spend the $9.8 million level 1 grant it had just been awarded (Michigan Senate Roll Call #675 2011). The House had approved a version of the bill a few weeks earlier, although its vote took place before the state had received the grant and thus did not include this money (Michigan House Roll Call #422 2011). When the bill came back to the House, leaders removed the $9.8 million federal grant out of opposition to Obamacare. Rather than block the entire appropriations bill right before the Christmas recess in order to save this $9.8 million, House members approved the $352 supplemental by a vote of 101–7 on December 13 (Michigan House Roll Call #570 2011). Faced with a similar choice the next day, the Senate voted 20–17 to approve the most recent House version (Michigan Senate Roll Call #792). The supplemental appropriations bill passed comfortably, but without any money for the state to spend on exchange planning.

The blocking of the level 1 establishment grant by the House gave opponents of an exchange their first major victory in Michigan. The Snyder administration was frustrated to lose this planning money. As one advisor put it, this was a "chicken and the egg sort of problem. If someone asked what our user fee would be in ten years, or something like that, I can't tell them . . . we needed their approval to get the funding to do this research" (Interview May 2013). But without answers to these questions, House Republicans were wary of voting to create an exchange.

January 19 House Health Policy Committee Hearing

This phase in the House debate over an insurance exchange culminated with a dramatic meeting of the House Health Policy Committee on January 19, 2012. Despite near-blizzard conditions and temperatures below 20°F, well more than one hundred people attended what was billed by Chairwoman Haines as an opportunity for public testimony. The meeting had to be moved from the regular committee room in the House Office Building to the ornate House Appropriations Committee Room on the third floor of the Capitol Building in order to accommodate the crowd. There were no presentations, no questions from committee members, and no scheduled vote. Instead, the committee listened for more than three hours as citizens and groups took turns giving three- to five-minute testimonies.

Tea Party activists were aggressive in mobilizing its members to attend (Gavette 2012; Fabiano 2012a). RightMichigan.com said, "a show of force sends the message that we do not want Obama Care (creation of a Health Care Exchange) and your presence also helps to support those in the House who oppose it" (Fabiano 2011b). Members of the Tea Party movement responded. The Lakes Area Tea Party had a table near the room's entrance containing literature against an exchange. Of the thirty-one people who testified, twenty were opposed. Of those, thirteen either identified themselves as being members of a Tea Party group or have an online presence at a Tea Party website.[3] Another twenty-one people emailed the committee clerk their testimony and forty-four submitted cards at the meeting but did not testify. Nearly half of the people sending emails sent a message that was exactly the same or a variation of a Tea Party form letter saying, "Please enter this email into the record. I am against *any* health care exchange in Michigan" (for example, see Iler 2012). A similar proportion of those submitting cards at the meeting identified themselves as being part of the Tea Party.

To put these numbers in perspective, a combined total of three people submitted cards during the first four meetings the committee held on an exchange the previous September and October. An earlier example of Tea Party mobilization occurred two months prior, on October 17, 2011. Fabiano called for the movement to engage in "focused activism" directed entirely at stopping SB 693. She wrote, "Attendance at a Committee

Meeting **is more effective than large rallies**. Most groups never achieve a 'tipping point' of attendance to influence Committee voting. Those that do create the buzz that puts the members of the committee, those testifying and the press on notice, that this is no ordinary meeting" (emphasis in the original, Fabiano 2012b). Thirteen people submitted cards opposing SB 693 at the next meeting, of which ten had an online presence on Tea Party websites (MI HHEAL 2011c). Only one person submitted cards at the next three meetings combined. In the first meeting after the Senate passed SB 693 and Tea Party activists issued another call to arms, of thirteen people who submitted cards against an exchange—eight were identified with the Tea Party (MI HHEAL 2011d). This meeting was a dramatic example of the Tea Party's ability to mobilize attendance at legislative meetings.

It was not just the number of the Tea Party activists in attendance at the January 19 meeting that was striking but also the content and tone of their arguments. Nearly one-third of the people who testified quoted articles produced by the Mackinac Center, either in part or in their entirety. They testified that creating an exchange was the same as implementing Obamacare. They argued that anyone who said Michigan did not have a choice or that an exchange would be happening anyway was either lying or uninformed. Multiple people compared the ACA to socialism. At least three people referenced Adolf Hitler and Nazi death camps in saying that creating an exchange puts the state on a dangerous path. One person referred at length to the Alfred Hitchcock movie *Psycho*—though it was not entirely clear why. Testimony by Tea Party activists was greeted with loud applause, whereas testimony in support of an exchange was almost always followed by silence.

It is hard to gauge what impact the Tea Party presence at this meeting had on SB 693's prospects in the House. Republican reactions were mixed, with Tea Party allies feeling emboldened and those outside the movement feeling frustrated. One Republican House staff member called the Tea Party activists attending this meeting "a fanatic sub-group of a party that has hijacked thinking" (Interview February 2012). Traditional stakeholder groups had a hard time knowing how to combat Tea Party arguments made at meetings like this. As one insurance leader described, "They will question everything you give them. The traditional things don't work. You can't just put out an argument and have them accept it. They will break it down" (Interview May 2013).

The decision to delay a vote until after the Supreme Court's ruling had already been made before the January 19 meeting (Interviews 2012–2013) and House Republicans had already blocked the $9.8 million level

1 establishment grant. However, now that the lines were clearly drawn in the sand, it would be very difficult for House Republicans to support an exchange should it come up for a vote.

The House Health Policy Committee continued to hold its regular meetings throughout 2012, though nobody brought up the issue of a health insurance exchange before June 28, when the Supreme Court ruling was announced. With support from Governor Snyder and passage in the Senate, supporters of an exchange now had the 20 and the 1. They would have to wait until the end of November before finding out whether they could also secure 56 votes in the House.

JULY 2012—OCTOBER 2013

The debate over a health insurance exchange during the fourth postenactment period progressed through three stages: (1) reacting to the Supreme Court's ruling by delaying making a decision until after the elections in November, (2) scrambling to decide once President Obama was reelected, and (3) trying to create a partnership exchange when the MI Health Marketplace failed.

Reaction to the Supreme Court

For nearly a year, opponents of creating a health insurance exchange in Michigan argued that it would not be prudent to act before the Supreme Court ruled on the constitutionality of the law. They said there would be plenty of time to move forward with plans to create an exchange if the ACA was upheld. As the ruling grew near, an increasing number of opponents argued that if the law survived, the state should actually wait until after the November election to decide. If it was struck down, then the state could move on and would be spared the work of creating an exchange. Supporters warned that the federal deadline by which states would have to declare their intention was November 16. This would give Michigan just ten days to pass authorizing legislation and prepare its application.

Reaction in Michigan to the Court's ruling was mixed, particularly in regard to what it would mean for the debate over an insurance exchange. Governor Snyder released a statement later that day expressing his dislike of the ACA as a law but argued it was time to pass legislation creating the MI Health Marketplace and to unfreeze the federal dollars from the $9.8 million level 1 grant (Snyder 2012a). Speaker Bolger wrote that he "could not be more upset" by the ruling, but that he would "work with Governor Snyder and the state Senate to see that Michiganders have access to health care that is marketplace-driven and provides competition, transparency, and common sense options. . . . A health care exchange is not something we wish to do, but we cannot stand idly by and hand over citizens' health care to an overreaching federal bureaucracy" (Thoms 2012). At least one Republican member of the House Health Policy Committee became convinced it was now time to act on SB 693. Representative Mike Callton of Nashville said that although he had favored waiting, he now feared the Republican Party was in danger of "focusing too much on ideology" and he would support an exchange (Skubick 2012a).

Attorney General Bill Schuette emerged as the most prominent Republican calling for the House to wait until after the election before making a decision (White, Mejia, and Clark 2012). Schuette's position as the state chairman for Republican presidential nominee Mitt Romney put Republicans who wanted to push for an exchange in a difficult position. Romney had a history of creating an exchange as governor of Massachusetts but opposed the creation of such exchanges under the ACA. Republican leaders worried that it would confuse the party's national narrative if a swing-state led by Republicans implemented a key component of Obamacare.

Shortly after Schuette's statement on waiting until the election, Speaker Bolger moderated his initial statement about an exchange, saying, "Having the state establish a healthcare exchange is not something we want to do" (Skubick 2012b). Gail Haines, chair of the House Health Policy Committee, responded in kind, saying, "We have taken a very prudent course up to this point and I see us taking the same course now" (Thoms 2012). Her committee did discuss the issue over the summer, though no vote was taken and no action was recommended (MI HHEAL 2012a). Tea Party leader Joan Fabiano wrote that she had spoken with Haines, who promised to continue "holding the fort" and not allow the appropriation of the $9.8 million federal grant (Fabiano 2012c).

Fabiano also warned that Governor Snyder might "try to be sneaky" and create an exchange by executive order (Fabiano 2012c). Governors in Rhode Island, Kentucky, and New York had already taken this path. Those close to the governor and legislative leadership say that this was never seriously considered, since he would need legislation to create an exchange as a nonprofit entity and that he was not interested in other governance structures (Interviews 2013). In any case, the legislature had demonstrated that it would not appropriate the money to fund an exchange, so creating an exchange by executive order would be futile. Given this set of circumstances, Snyder and other supporters had no choice but to wait until after the election before trying again.

SB 693 Fails in Lame Duck Session

Governor Snyder gave a speech to the House Republican Caucus behind closed doors shortly after President Obama won reelection and it became apparent the ACA would be implemented. According to someone in the room, he compared the ACA to a "speeding train coming at you. You can either jump off the tracks and just let it go past you and hope it won't destroy everything you built behind you, or you can jump on the train and do your best to have some controls to transform it as best as possible." Not everyone agreed. Some responded that it was not their train and they did not set it in motion. If it crashes, let the federal government be blamed for it, not the states (Interview May 2013). Yet by this point, Speaker Bolger and Chairwoman Haines had evolved and were among those pushing for passage of SB 693.

With the November 16 deadline ten days away, it seemed that there was not enough time to act. The Obama administration faced a dilemma about whether to hold firm to its deadlines and let states deal with the consequence of a federal takeover or to relax deadlines and continue to encourage states to take control of their exchange. HHS had already extended the deadline for the level 2 establishment grant from what turned out to be the day after the Supreme Court issued its ruling until 2014. The administration made a similar decision with the November 16 deadline, giving states until December 14. It then gave states choosing not to run their own exchange until February 15 to submit plans to create a partnership. After the extensions, Speaker Bolger published a letter forcefully calling for a state-based exchange. He wrote:

> The question as to whether there will be an exchange in Michigan is now answered by the courts and the voters: there will be an exchange. The question we need to answer is whether the state will have a seat at that table, or if we will cede state control to the federal government and allow them to establish the exchange with federal priorities rather than Michigan priorities. Michigan can assert its sovereign rights and responsibilities to protect its citizens to minimize federal overreach.

Bolger further argued that a federal exchange would have limited choice, whereas an exchange run by Michigan would be open, religious liberties would be protected, and the state could ensure that agents and brokers play a role as navigators. Finally, he warned that a federally run exchange would be a slippery slope toward a single-payer system (Bolger 2012).

Extensions on deadlines gave states with year-round legislatures a second chance. Ironically, federal flexibility on deadlines also emboldened opponents to further resist an exchange. Business leaders and consumer advocates in Michigan say they heard many opponents question why they should believe HHS on anything since they continued to give in (Interviews 2012–2013). Opponents believed HHS lacked the will and the capacity to create three dozen exchanges simultaneously and that the whole effort would fail if enough states resisted. Continued flexibility on the part of federal officials gave credibility to these arguments.

Within a week of Speaker Bolger's letter, Chairwoman Haines announced that her committee would hold a vote on SB 693 during its meeting on November 29. Republican staff members give conflicting reports about whether leadership was convinced it had enough votes to get the bill through committee. Some say they had verbal commitments from enough people. Others say that legislators had been entrenched for so long "that there was no wiggle room" (Interviews 2012–2013). Even if the votes were not secured ahead of the meeting, Snyder and other leaders felt it was time for closure. Agency bureaucrats at the state and federal levels needed to know what the plan would be for preparing for open enrollment beginning in October 2013. As one Republican House staff member put it, "Our thought was to put it up, see what happens. If it passes, then we'll work like the dickens to get the vote on the floor. If not, then we move to plan B" (Interview May 2013).

The tension of the January 29 meeting was still in people's minds as they heard presentations from agency officials, as well as testimony from ten people from the audience and received position cards from twenty-six people. The public attending the hearing was evenly split, with half of the people voicing an opinion in support SB 693 and half opposing. According to a comment on RightMichigan.com, more than seven hundred emails opposing SB 693 were sent to legislators leading up to the meeting (Heine 2012).

The bill's defeat at this meeting on November 29 was described by some participants as a perfect storm of multiple factors (Interviews 2012–2013). Exchange politics became entangled with political battles over other contentious issues. Proposals to enact "Right to Work" legislation against unions in the lame duck session were gaining momentum, with some Republicans nervously remembering the outcry over this issue the year before in Wisconsin. Democrats threatened to vote against all Republican bills as a way to gain leverage in the Right to Work debate, meaning Democrats might vote against SB 693 after calling for its passage for a year.

According to one staff member, Chairwoman Haines made a deal with Republican members of the committee that she would tie-bar the exchange to two other bills (HB 4143 and HB 4147), which would prohibit qualified health plans from paying for elective abortions. This means that even if the House approved SB 693 and it was signed by the governor, an exchange would not be authorized until these two abortion-related bills were also passed. Apparently not everyone was aware of this deal and the meeting had to be recessed twice as both sides deliberated how to proceed. One business leader described this as a "really strange time" in which "things got weird" (Interview May 2013).

Democrats had been freed by leadership to vote for an exchange instead of maintain the Right to Work boycott, though some were not sure they still wanted to, given the abortion connection. Representative Marcia Hovey-Wright (D), who was the National Organization of Women's Michigan Chapter Legislator of the Year, proposed eliminating the tie-bar. Her motion failed 12 to 4, with Representative George Darany (D) abstaining (Gautz 2012). The exchange bill the committee had been considering for more than a year was now also suddenly a bill about access to abortion, complicating the calculus for Democratic members of the committee.

The final vote was nine opposed to creating an exchange and five in favor, with two abstaining, one not registering a vote, and two being absent (Table 3.2). This vote effectively killed SB 693 and Michigan's prospect of running its own exchange. The bill was much closer to passage than this tally makes it appear and may have passed had it not been connected to abortion. Representative Mike Callton was the only Republican other than Chairwoman Haines to vote in favor of an exchange. The abortion connection may have made it easier for him to cast this vote, but he had already expressed support for an exchange and may well have voted for SB 693 in any case (Interviews 2013). Democrat Representatives Hovey-Wright and Segal both voted "pass," meaning they abstained, but they had supported an exchange and likely would have voted in favor of SB 693 had it not been tie-barred to abortion.

If these two Democrats had voted in favor, and if the two absent Democrats had shown up for the meeting and voted with the rest of their party as their earlier comments suggest they would have, this would have brought the vote to a 9–9 tie. It is not clear why these members were absent—they did not respond to inquiries for a comment. Representative Jimmy Womack (D) had been robbed at gunpoint near his home in Detroit a few months earlier, but was unharmed in the incident (Burns 2012). Instead, Womack stopped attending meetings after losing his primary race in August. Womack was not a regular attendee of his committee meetings

Table 3.2. HOUSE HEALTH POLICY COMMITTEE ROLL CALL ON SB 693, NOVEMBER 29, 2012

Voting Yes (5)
Gail Haines, R—Committee Chair
Mike Callton, R—Majority Vice-Chair
George Darany, D
Tim Greimel, D
Thomas Stallworth, D
Voting No (9)
Joseph Graves, R
Tom Hooker, R
Holly Hughes, R
Matt Huuki, R
Ken Kurtz, R
Paul Muxlow, R
Paul Opsommer, R
Mike Shirkey, R
Ken Yonker, R
Voting "Pass" (3)
Wayne Schmidt, 3
Marcia Hovey-Wright, D
Kate Segal, D
Absent (2)
Lesia Liss, D—Minority Vice-Chair
Jimmy Womack, D

anyway, missing 75% of the hearings on a health insurance exchange.[4] After the electoral loss, he stopped attending hearings altogether, missing every meeting of his three committee assignments between August and December 2012.[5]

Representative Lesia Liss (D) was the other Democrat not to show. This was noteworthy, given her role as the minority vice-chair on the committee and that this was her first time not attending a hearing on the exchange. Republican staff members speculate that she did not want to join Democrats in the blockade they were considering of all Republican bills and expected that SB 693 would be defeated anyway (Interviews 2012–2013). Liss had a troubled relationship with her caucus, particularly on abortion issues (Baerren 2012), and had just been defeated in the August primaries. But unlike Womack, she continued to come to Lansing after her defeat; two days earlier she attended a meeting of the Military and Veterans Affairs and Homeland Security Committee (HMILI 2012). It is interesting to note that the November 29 Health Policy meeting was the first time someone on the committee did not make a motion to excuse the members who were absent (HHEAL 2012b). Ironically, almost half the time it had been Representative Liss who made that motion.

Assuming Representative Callton would have maintained his support for SB 693, and Representatives Segal and Hovey-Wright would have voted in favor without the tie-bar, and if the two absent Democrats showed up and voted with their caucus, Representative Wayne Schmidt would have been the deciding vote. The exchange was not an easy issue for him. During the Republican primary a few months earlier, Americans for Prosperity sent out a flyer with Schmidt's face alongside pictures of Democratic leaders Nancy Pelosi, Barack Obama, and Harry Reid. Surrounding these pictures were the words "Will your representative Wayne Schmidt be an Obamacare collaborator . . . or will he oppose building its infrastructure in Michigan?" (Gillman 2012). At a primary debate in Traverse City, he refused to sign a pledge against creating an exchange, saying "I've opposed instituting Obamacare, and I'm still not in favor of it . . . but the Supreme Court has ruled. It's my job and my fellow legislators' job to do what is best for the people of the state of Michigan" (McGillivary 2012). If he would have followed through with this tepid support of an exchange, then the committee would have approved the bill 10-9.

A Republican staff member described the November 2012 committee vote saying, "This was not a vote against a state-based exchange or a vote for a federal exchange, but a vote against doing something with too many unanswered questions" (Interview December 2012). An advisor to Governor Snyder feels they could have won approval of SB 693 if they had the answer to more of the questions that were asked about how the exchange would operate and that they could have had these answers if the federal government had been faster at issuing regulations (Interview May 2013). An insurance leader commented, "The more doubt you have, the harder it is. The longer it took to get the regs out, the more it fed people's doubts" (Interview May 2013). Flexibility by HHS ironically made a vote on SB 693 possible, but undermined its likelihood of passage.

The split within the Republican Party made it difficult for the Snyder administration to win enough support. They had to reach out to Democrats to get the necessary 56 votes in the House and 20 votes in the Senate, though this made it more difficult to gain support from conservatives. The more conservative wing of the Republican Party was unsure of Governor Snyder, given that he won office because of his status as an outsider. Efforts at bipartisanship were met with suspicion by conservatives. Some said that they did not know very much about the issue, but there must be reason to be concerned if Democrats were willing to work with Governor Snyder (Interviews 2011–2013). As one conservative leader put it, "Bi-partisanship is a fallacy. It's impossible when you come from polar opposite philosophies without completely abdicating your positions. It's impossible" (Interview May 2013).

Tea Party members warned lawmakers that the future of the American republic was at stake over the exchange vote. They felt a responsibility to be loud, given what they perceived as the high stakes. When asked whether the Obama or Snyder administrations could have done anything that would have won their support of health reform, one prominent Tea Party activist responded "No, because it's really the antithesis of our form of government." This person further replied, "These types of things need to be addressed on a state and local level. I concur that there needs to be a reform in insurance, but it should be done at the state level and open to private market solutions" (Interview May 2013). They refused to consider that this was the goal of the state-based insurance exchange supported by Governor Snyder.

The Tea Party successfully created a climate in which it was difficult for Republican lawmakers to support an exchange. This was particularly true in the House, where there was a greater concentration of Tea Party strength than in the Senate. Of the nine Republicans on the House Health Policy Committee who voted against SB 693, all but three had a Tea Party rating greater than 70%. Two members of the committee were in the top ten in terms of Tea Party rating (Michiganvotes 2012). It would have been very difficult for these legislators to support an exchange given the Tea Party's large presence on the issue. Interest groups on the other side of the issue could have promised to support Republican legislators who bucked the Tea Party on this issue, but seemed unwilling to do so. For example, representatives of Blue Cross Blue Shield of Michigan, the company with the largest share of the state's insurance market, explained that although they preferred state control, they were preparing along parallel paths to be ready either way. They had other important issues coming before the legislature soon and did not want to expend all their political capital on the exchange. This gave the Tea Party and conservative groups a greater opening to block the exchange bill.

Even so, House leadership was confident SB 693 would have passed had it reached the floor. As one senior staff member described, "Normally we don't try to ignore the Republican majority and try to pass things with the Democrats, but on an issue like this we would have. We would have lost some Republicans, but kept enough to add to the Democrats" (Interview May 2013).

Opponents of an exchange reacted with excitement to SB 693's defeat in committee. Jason Gillman wrote on RightMichigan.com, "Thanks, again conservative warriors. You are the modern day Minutemen!" (Gillman 2012). Tea Party activist Joan Fabiano wrote, "The Michigan Health Care Exchange bill was defeated in Committee! This is a victory for the grassroots, it's your victory" (Fabiano 2012d).

Technically, the bill was not actually dead. After the 5–9 vote, Representative Callton moved to reconsider the vote at a later date. The motion passed without objection. This gave the committee the option of revisiting the bill before the end of the year and taking another vote without having to introduce a new bill and start the process over in both chambers. This motion gave supporters of an exchange a sliver of hope, though Speaker Bolger quickly announced that although he would have preferred a state-based exchange, the issue would not be brought up again during this session (Gautz 2012). With that statement from the Speaker, it was official that after more than two years of debate, Michigan would not be creating its own exchange. The Snyder administration said they would work to take over control of the state's exchange in its second or third year. In the meantime, their focus shifted to establishing a partnership exchange (Snyder 2012b).

Partnership Funds Approved by House, Blocked by Senate

LARA submitted its second level 1 establishment grant application by November 15. This application was to support the creation of a partnership exchange even though it was still two weeks before the House Health Policy Committee voted to block a state-run exchange. At least one legislative staff member felt it sent a mixed message to House Republicans that the governor was working so hard on a contingency plan at the same that he was asking them to vote on a state-based exchange (Interview December 2012). An advisor to Governor Snyder responded that it was their responsibility to do everything possible to be prepared in either case (Interview May 2013). The new grant was broad so that it could be used if the state moved forward with its own exchange, but also specifically addressed the planning activities that the Snyder administration would focus on in a partnership, such as plan management and consumer assistance (CMS 2014). When SB 693 died in committee, this grant became the basis for the state's application to run a partnership exchange with CMS.

The federal government awarded Michigan its $30.7 million level 1 grant on January 17, 2013 (CMS 2014), giving the state a month before the new February 15 deadline to submit a letter of intent and partnership blueprint. Within a week, Governor Snyder sent a letter to Secretary Sebelius declaring intention to create a partnership exchange (Snyder 2013). A blueprint was submitted shortly after that, with conditional approval given by HHS on March 5. To receive full approval, Michigan would have to: (1) demonstrate the ability to perform the exchange functions; (2) comply with regulations and expected progress milestones, (3) sign a memorandum of understanding between LARA and the Medicaid agency defining the roles, responsibilities, and coordinated work by each agency; and (4) demonstrate legal and spending authority for exchange activities (Sebelius 2013). The first three points were within reach, though the fourth proved to be the undoing of the partnership.

The legislature did not need to approve the governor's plan for a partnership exchange, but it did need to authorize any money that would be spent to create and implement such an exchange. The interest groups supporting an exchange were optimistic the legislature would approve the funds for three reasons. First, they noted that the House was more moderate in 2013 than in the previous two years, with the Republican margin having been reduced in half by the 2012 elections (Interviews 2013). As a result, interest groups felt Republican lawmakers responded to lobbying on an exchange with less resistance, perhaps even supporting a transition to state control in future years. As one person put it, "part of this came from a feeling that the deadlines were real this time and that the federal government was not going to blink anymore" (Interview May 2013). Second, this time Speaker Bolger was pushing for passage with rank and file members saying things like, "I don't support Obamacare, but I don't have Obamacarephobia whereby I think that it's just going to go away if we do nothing" (Eggert 2013). Third, some of the opposition to an exchange was softening. On November 27, the NFIB released the results of a poll that found that although only 46% of its members supported creating a state-based exchange prior to the November election, it was now preferred by 73% (NFIB 2012). In this changed environment, the House Appropriations Committee approved the supplemental funding bill (Michigan House Bill [HB] 4111 2013) on February 27 by a vote of 24–3. The next day, nearly half (29/59) of the Republican House caucus voted with all but one Democrat to pass the bill on the floor 78–31. It seemed that the most difficult hurdle had been overcome.

Over the course of the two and a half year debate, the Senate had already voted to create a state-based exchange and to appropriate the original $9.8 million level 1 grant, leading stakeholders to assume it would do the same with latest grant. They did not lobby the Senate as aggressively as they had the House (Interviews 2013). On the other hand, Republican staffers describe this period as another awakening for conservative groups, particularly Americans for Prosperity, the Mackinac Center, and the Tea Party. As one House staff member put it, "I never saw the likes of the conservative groups come out until we passed the partnership money. It's like their heads came out of the sand when the issue came to us, but it was an all-out war in the Senate once we passed it." Enough Senators were sympathetic to their arguments and were responsive when these groups pointed out that each Senator would be up for reelection for the first time since 2010 and that their support was not guaranteed.

Senators felt burned by the House from the previous session's debate over SB 693 when they had stuck their neck out on a controversial vote only to have it ignored by the other chamber. They described their initial votes as being for state control, not to work side by side with President Obama, particularly as his "partner." Not only did they find this nuance difficult to explain to their constituents, they did not believe it would be a true partnership, since the federal government would dictate the terms. They feared this would make Michigan merely the complaint office for a federally run exchange (Interviews 2013).

The Senate never took a vote on HB 4111 to appropriate this $31 million level 1 grant. The Senate killed the possibility of a partnership exchange by letting federal deadlines pass without authorizing the state to spend this money on planning activities. House leaders thought Governor Snyder might push for approval of this funding during the annual budget negotiations later that spring, but he did not (Interview May 2013). When the Michigan exchange began operating on January 1, 2014, it was not run by the state or as a partnership, but was part of the federal exchange.

CHAPTER 4

Idaho

INTRODUCTION

Idaho is an unlikely candidate for the distinction of being the only state in the nation led by a Republican governor and a Republican legislature to run its health insurance exchange. Public opinion polling and measures used by political scientists suggest it is one of the most conservative states in the country (Shor and McCarty 2011).[1] Idahoans voted for the Republican nominee in every presidential election since 1964, including giving Barack Obama only 36% of the vote in 2008 and 32% in 2012 (see Table 4.1). Since 1981, both US senators have been Republicans. With one brief exception from 2009 to 2010, both of Idaho's US representatives have been Republicans since 1995. State government is similarly dominated by Republicans. Idahoans have not elected a Democratic governor in two decades and have consistently elected large Republican majorities in both chambers of the legislature.

Most of Idaho's leaders opposed the Affordable Care Act. All four members of the state's congressional delegation voted against the law, including Democrat Walt Minnick. Idaho was the first state in the nation to enact legislation opposing the ACA, even before President Obama signed the bill into law in March 2010 (CBS News 2010). Idaho was also among the first states to sue the federal government over the constitutionality of the ACA. The dominant interest groups in the state were nearly unanimous in their opposition to the ACA.

Table 4.1. IDAHO'S POLITICAL AND DEMOGRAPHIC CONTEXT

Political Environment

- 2012 presidential election: Mitt Romney (65%)
- Governor
  - 2007–present: C. L. "Butch" Otter (R)
  - No term limits
- Idaho House of Representatives
  - 2011–2012: Republican majority of forty-four
  - 2013–2015: Republican majority of forty-four
  - No term limits
- Idaho Senate
  - 2011–2012: Republican majority of twenty-one
  - 2013–2015: Republican majority of twenty-three
  - No term limits

Demographics & Health Status

- Total population: 1,580,000
- Distribution of Population by Federal Poverty Level
  - Under 100%: 19%
  - 100%–138%: 10%
  - 139%–399%: 45%
  - 400%: 27%
- Distribution of Health Insurance Coverage
  - Employer: 47%
  - Other private: 7%
  - Medicaid: 14%
  - Medicare: 15%
  - Uninsured: 16%

Health Reform

- Joined lawsuit against the ACA
- State-based exchange, relying on national website for first year
- Not expanding Medicaid

Three years later, many of the same leaders who had opposed the ACA pushed for the state to take control over the implementation of an insurance exchange. Why did Idaho choose this path? What happened between March 2010, when the state's leaders were united against the ACA, and March 2013, when Governor C. L. "Butch" Otter successfully pushed for the creation of a state-based insurance exchange?

There were many twists along the way, including the rejection of federal grants, nullification bills, a veto, and an executive order. Ultimately, the issue split the Republican caucus with enough joining the Democrats to support an exchange. Prominent interest groups worked hard to support state control, though not without strong opposition from the Tea Party and conservative groups. Four factors emerge as particularly significant in Idaho: (1) Governor Otter's strong support, (2) the development of a strong industry coalition, (3) the support and influence of key legislative leaders, and (4) moments not directly connected to the exchange debate that empowered some people at the expense of others (see Appendix C for a timeline of key events in Idaho).

MARCH 2010—DECEMBER 2010

The initial months of the ACA's implementation in Idaho were marked by sharp opposition to the law. The events of this period laid the foundation for the debate that would follow in subsequent years, including the passage of the Idaho Health Freedom Act, the multistate lawsuit against the ACA's mandates, the growth of the Tea Party, and the creation of the conservative think tank the Idaho Freedom Foundation (IFF). Yet even in a period notable for hostility toward the reform as a whole, the Otter administration took steps behind the scenes to begin implementing an exchange.

Idaho Health Freedom Act

The state's response to the Affordable Care Act began before the ACA was signed into law. In his state of the state speech on January 11, 2010, Governor Otter spoke in opposition to "the so-called health care 'reform' bills being promoted by the President's party in Congress." He warned that an expansion of Medicaid would cost the state half a billion dollars and thanked the Idaho congressional delegation for "fighting against this wholesale assault on our self-determination" (Otter 2010).

Republicans in the state legislature were similarly opposed. On January 19, Representatives Jim Clark, Raul Labrador, and Lynn Luker introduced House Bill 391, which they named the Idaho Health Freedom Act. In the words of a lobbyist for a major business organization, the act was a preemptive measure "to tell the federal government that we'll stay in charge of our health care and you stay out of it" (Interview May 2013). The likelihood of the ACA's passage was coincidentally seriously jeopardized later that same day, as Massachusetts Republican Scott Brown won the special election to fill Ted Kennedy's seat in the US Senate. As a result, Democrats no longer had a filibuster-proof majority and many considered health reform dead (see chapter 1 for more details).

The Idaho Health Freedom Act was based on model legislation developed by the national organization the American Legislative Exchange Council (ALEC) (News on 6 2010). HB 391 stated that the US Constitution's 9th and 10th amendments limit the role of the federal government in healthcare, and established, "every person within the state of Idaho is and shall be free to choose or decline any mode of securing health care services without penalty or threat of penalty." In other words, the bill asserted that the individual mandate being considered by Congress is not constitutional and would not be in effect in Idaho. No public official or agent of the state would be allowed to play any role in such a mandate. HB 391 also directed the state's attorney general to respond promptly to any federal law that challenged the state's role as defined in this bill (Idaho House Bill [ID HB] 391 2010).

The Republican leadership prioritized the Idaho Health Freedom Act, moving it quickly through the legislative process, even as the national reform remained in limbo. It was one of the first bills introduced in the session and only the second bill to receive a hearing by the Senate State Affairs Committee. The bill was amended to clarify that although the government would not be allowed to mandate that everyone purchase insurance, it would still be legal for the state to require that college and university students obtain coverage. Republican Senator Monty Pearce, who ultimately voted for the Idaho Health Freedom Act, said the amended bill looks hypocritical in that it rails against a federal mandate but specifically protects one by the state. Republican Representative Clark, one of the bill's sponsors, responded that mandates may be good ideas sometimes, but that it is the state's right to experiment.

The bill passed the House completely along party lines and then passed the Senate with all but three Republicans voting in favor. Governor Otter signed the bill on March 17, four days before the ACA passed the US House and a week before it passed the US Senate and was signed into law by President Obama. Governor Otter felt the issue was important enough for his first public bill signing ceremony of the 2010 session. In the press conference that followed, Governor Otter spoke strongly against the federal health reform. Ironically using many of the same arguments he would later use to defend his support of a state-based health insurance exchange, Governor Otter stated that HB 391 was important because it asserted the sovereignty of the state (Hurst 2010a).

The passage of the Idaho Health Freedom Act was a significant opening shot in the battle over the ACA's implementation in Idaho. Governor Otter and the legislature staked a position in strong opposition to the reform and in support of the joint lawsuit that Attorney General Wasden filed with Florida and eleven other states minutes after President Obama signed the ACA into law. Interest groups had their first opportunity to weigh in on what the law would mean for Idaho, with the American Association for Retired Persons (AARP) testifying against the bill (and thus for the ACA), the Idaho Farm Bureau testifying in favor, and the Idaho Republican Central Committee passing a parallel resolution against the ACA (Idaho [ID] Senate State Affairs Committee 2010).

One of the most important developments during this time was the growing role of the IFF. Formed in 2009, the IFF is a nonprofit organization led by Wayne Hoffman, a former journalist and staff member to Idaho politicians. Hoffman describes the passage of the Idaho Health Freedom Act as one of his group's earliest accomplishments (Russell 2010). In just a few short years, the IFF would be considered one of the most influential and controversial groups in the state. It would play a lead role in the debate over the ACA's implementation in Idaho, making opposing the exchange and Medicaid two of its top legislative priorities.

2010 Elections and the Growth of the Tea Party

As the legislature passed the Idaho Health Freedom Act it was unclear what effect the law would have. Attorney General Wasden did not need the legislature's permission to file a lawsuit, and it would be up to the courts to decide whether the federal government had the authority to impose mandates, not state legislatures. Deputy Attorney General Jones admitted to the Senate State Affairs Committee that federal law would likely trump the Idaho legislature on this issue, raising questions about the legal validity of this bill. Even so, HB 391 was hugely important symbolically, as 2010 was an election year, with the Republican primaries less than two months after the close of the legislative session at the end of March. Republican incumbents and challengers used their support of the Idaho Health Freedom Act to validate their conservative credentials.

The most prominent example is Raul Labrador, who had been one of the bill's sponsors and ran for the 1st district seat in the US House on a platform that included repealing the ACA. Organizations such as Idaho Chooses Life specifically cited his work opposing health reform as the reason for their endorsement (Hurst 2010b). Labrador won a surprise victory in the May 2010 Republican primary, beating Vaughn Ward, who had been one of the top ten candidates in the National Republican Congressional Committee's Young Guns recruiting program and was endorsed by Sarah Palin (Blake 2010).

Labrador's victory in the primary set up an interesting general election contest against Walt Minnick, who was among the most conservative Democrats in Congress and who had voted against the ACA (Hulse 2010). The race was complicated by the fact that in April 2010 the national Tea Party Express had endorsed Walt Minnick for reelection. This was the first election cycle since the inception of the Tea Party in 2009, and it was unclear whether their involvement would be consequential. Minnick was the only Democrat in the country to receive an endorsement from the Tea Party Express, and his campaign worried it would hurt him with Democrats and moderates. Three months after tepidly accepting the endorsement in April 2010, Minnick rejected it in July (Stein 2010). By the fall, the Tea Party Express endorsed Labrador and was running ads accusing Minnick of becoming more liberal the longer he stays in Congress. Even though he voted just a few months earlier against the ACA, they lambasted him for refusing to advocate for its repeal (Tea Party Express 2010). At the end of the summer, Labrador was losing by thirty points and had only $69,000 in the bank compared to Minnick's $1.1 million (Ames 2011). With the support of Tea Party groups across the state, Labrador beat Minnick 51%–41% in the general election. He went on to become a prominent national figure in the evolution of the Tea Party in Congress.

Labrador's success was an indication of the prominent role that the Tea Party could play in Idaho politics and generated momentum that would be important in subsequent legislative sessions. At this point, the Tea Party was a decentralized but active network of organizations spread across the state. Pam Stout, leader of the Tea Party organization in Sandpoint in northern Idaho, made an appearance on the *David Letterman Show* and was described in the *New York Times* as being "the hub of a rapidly expanding and highly viral network" (Barstow 2010). Skocpol and Williamson's (2012) survey of the Tea Party in 2011 found that Idaho is one of only seven states to have as many as four to six Tea Party organizations per million residents but not have a single city with more than five hundred registered members. One online directory of Tea Party organizations lists thirteen groups throughout the state (Tea Party 911 2013), while another lists fifteen (Gem State Tea Party 2013). It was unclear whether these groups could be mobilized in a coordinated way, but this election showed their potential influence.

Labrador's victory was also an indication of the level of discontent Idahoans felt for the health reform law. Opposing the ACA would not be enough to prevent attacks from conservatives and the Tea Party. Candidates needed to demonstrate the intensity of their dislike for the law, including pushing for its repeal. Campaigning on a platform of opposing the implementation of Obamacare in Idaho, Governor Otter was reelected and Republicans retained large majorities in the 2010 elections, winning 80% of the seats in the Senate and 74% of the seats in the House. Though the partisan margins remained similar, the legislature moved further to the right, with a handful of seats in Republican districts going to the most conservative candidate rather than a moderate. The legislature that would be considering the ACA's implementation during the crucial years of 2011 and 2012 was therefore even more conservative than the legislature that passed the Idaho Health Freedom Act.

Workgroups and Planning Grants

As legislators pushed for the ACA's repeal, work was being done behind the scenes to prepare for its implementation. Two agencies played a lead role in this process: the Department of Insurance focused on the exchanges, while the Department of Health and Welfare focused on the Medicaid expansion. An official at the Department of Insurance describes the dilemma faced by the department:

> All of us key decision makers in Idaho did not want the ACA passed. There were a lot of credible reasons as to why it did not need to be passed. Our congressional delegation and local legislators all agree that this wasn't the right choice to make health care available to more people. At the same time, we probably didn't have a better idea, but we had a better idea how we could do it in Idaho, with the help of federal dollars, to get this turned around in Idaho. (Interview May 2013)

The dilemma was all the more pronounced, given that Governor Otter and Insurance Commissioner Bill Deal had already created a health insurance exchange on a smaller scale. Shortly after taking office in 2007, Governor Otter had convened a task force to improve the affordability and accessibility of healthcare in Idaho. One of the recommendations was to establish a website on which consumers could compare the products of the three main insurance companies. Legislation was not sought, but in subsequent months a simple and small-scale shopping page was added to the Department of Insurance website.

An insurance department official explains that Deal and the Otter administration were not opposed to an exchange in principle, but saw Obamacare's version as overly cumbersome (Interview May 2013). Even so, their initial reaction was to explore what it would mean to build their own ACA-compliant exchange so that they did not have to give up control to the federal government. On September 30, 2010, Idaho was one of forty-eight states awarded a planning grant by the Centers for Medicare and Medicaid Services (CMS). The state received $1 million to accomplish ten tasks, including "engage stakeholders and create strategies for continued engagement," "evaluate existing government and non-government structures for opportunities to integrate these structures to support an exchange," "create recommendations for governance structures," and "identify needed enabling legislation and regulations" (CMS 2014).

Although primarily focused on Medicaid, the Department of Health and Welfare played an important role in the planning for an exchange. In 2009, the department had begun implementing a new Medicaid eligibility system for the first time in twenty years. As one official described it, the new Medicaid system would have to connect with whatever exchange was created, whether by the state or the federal government. "It didn't matter which kind of exchange it was; we have a new friend in town we need to work with" (Interview October 2013). This new IT system would ultimately become an important component of the eligibility determination process of Idaho's exchange.

Officials in both agencies describe the difficulty of preparing for the ACA's implementation given the state's political climate, particularly with a governor and legislature so firmly opposed to the law. One Medicaid official explained:

> We were trying to figure out how to do this without upsetting anybody and make them think we're going against anybody. Our approach is saying that this is the law of the land, what do you expect us to do? If we don't meet the law and timelines, there are consequences funding-wise, especially for Medicaid. You can't say we have a choice—we have to connect to an exchange. (Interview October 2013)

Compounding the challenge was the fact that leaders in the agencies felt they were not getting enough direction from the Obama administration. They resisted federal involvement, but also feared they would have to retrace their steps once CMS finally issued regulations. Another bureaucrat said, "We went pretty fast to try and get this moved, and I think federal agencies were scrambling to try and catch up and do it in a way that is meaningful to states. . . . It got pretty old pretty quickly to continually be told 'we'll get back to you' by CMS" (Interview October 2013).

In December 2010, Governor Otter followed through with a commitment in the state's planning grant to engage stakeholders on the ACA's implementation. He issued an executive order calling for the creation of the Idaho Health Care Council comprising agency officials and stakeholders appointed by the governor. The three workgroups that were created became an important forum for stakeholders to voice their opinions on the ACA. Ultimately, the seeds for the creation of a state-based exchange were sown in these meetings.

This was a delicate balancing act for the Otter administration. The Idaho Health Freedom Act passed earlier in 2010 said no state official was to play any role in implementing or enforcing a federal mandate. Some argued that bureaucrats were breaking this law by doing any work to prepare for the creation of an exchange and expansion of Medicaid. Settling this question would be one of the primary issues of the upcoming legislative session.

JANUARY 2011—OCTOBER 2011

The ACA had been signed into law by President Obama just two weeks before the close of Idaho's 2010 legislative session, meaning that 2011 was the first opportunity for the legislature to fully respond to the requirements of implementing health reform. Governor Otter's state of the state speech to open the session on January 10 struck a strong but balanced tone. He railed against "the exorbitant costs being imposed on us by Obamacare," and said he was working aggressively to eliminate the law either in the courts or through Congress. He specifically mentioned nullification—the idea that a state can declare a particular federal law null and void within its borders—as an option Idaho should consider. At the same time, he said, "we are responsibly preparing for watershed changes that may be on the way" (Otter 2011a). The 2011 legislative session was marked by tension between those pushing for nullification and those pushing for a state role in implementing the ACA.

Nullification

In the closing months of 2010 and the opening months of 2011, nullification legislation was introduced in at least thirteen states, including a bill with Governor Otter's support in Idaho. The attorney general's office, the same team that was in the midst of suing the federal government over the ACA, was not convinced, responding, "there is no right to pick and choose which federal laws a state will follow."

Wayne Hoffman of the IFF worked with legislators on the nullification bill, and the Tea Party mobilized large groups to attend committee hearings. They used many of the arguments that would later be made against doing an exchange, such as that Obamacare put the country on a dangerous path toward socialism. They also pointed to the debate about a national identification card—named REAL ID—as precedent that the federal government would delay enforcement of a mandate if enough states resisted.

The Idaho House approved the state's initial nullification proposal (HB 117) mostly along party lines, but the bill was defeated by the Senate State Affairs Committee after a volatile meeting. Audience members yelled out of turn in opposition to the ACA. Republican lawmakers who had just defeated the nullification bill were confronted by a Tea Party group standing outside the Senate auditorium accusing them of being cowards (Associated Press [AP] 2011a).

The fight over nullification did not die with these votes, as two more bills were introduced that session. One of them, HB 298, passed the House with similar margins as the previous bill and then made it through the Senate on a vote of 24–11. The goal of this bill was not to nullify the ACA per se, but to say that nobody in the state would be allowed to do anything related to its implementation. One Senate leader who voted against the original nullification bill but voted for HB 298 and would ultimately support a state-based exchange explained the bill this way:

> What we said to the opponents was, look, we'll take the governor's bill and take out the heavy-handed, we know it's not going anywhere, crap. We did not insert any new language, we just pulled out the obvious stuff and sent [Governor Otter] his bill, which was nullification-lite. It says we're not nullifying it, it's still law, but you can't force us to do it. The state of Idaho isn't going to do it; you're going to have to do it. (Interview April 2013)

Two weeks later, Governor Otter vetoed HB 298, his only veto of the 2011 legislative session. The same Senator who had supported the bill described being stunned, wanting to say to Governor Otter, "What do you mean we can't do this? This is your bill! It's your bill, less the nullification stuff!" (Interview April 2013). The veto message began with a defense of Otter's conservative credentials, noting, "No one has opposed Obamacare more vehemently than me" and then reiterating his support for the previous year's Idaho Health Freedom Act and the multistate lawsuit of which Idaho was a part. The first explanation he gives for his veto was that it would eliminate the possibility that Idaho would be able to create a health insurance exchange. He clarified that he did not want to implement Obamacare, but that he also did not want to cede control to the federal government should all the avenues of opposition prove fruitless. He went on to write, "I see value in evaluating an Idaho Health Insurance Exchange and have been an advocate for doing so before the concept was co-opted by the national government" (Otter 2011b).

On the same day as his veto, Governor Otter issued Executive Order 2011-03 (2011) to accomplish many of the same objectives as HB 298 but still preserve the option of creating an exchange. State agencies were prevented from working on any aspect of implementing the ACA except planning for an exchange. One of Governor Otter's advisers explained, "Our office felt that the legislature didn't understand how deeply their bill would affect our state. The ACA has a lot of other parts the legislature's bill would have made much too difficult" (Interview June 2011). In addition to wanting to preserve the option of doing an exchange, Medicaid officials described wanting to take advantage of ACA grants to support upgrades to the state's eligibility system that were being done even before the ACA entered the picture (Interview October 2013).

Governor Otter was trying to walk a fine line between opposing the ACA and maintaining the option of state control of an exchange. Many conservatives wished he had gone further in his opposition, but were pleased with his executive order. The press release from the governor's office about the executive order included supportive quotes from people who would be his most ardent opponents on the exchange two years later. Wayne Hoffman of the IFF is described as having "worked closely with legislative sponsors of House Bill 298," but saw the executive order as "an important step in the right direction for Idaho and for freedom." Senator Russ Fulcher, who would challenge Otter for the Republican nomination for governor in 2014, largely over their difference on the exchange, was described as "welcoming" the executive order, saying, "I'm just thankful to have the Governor's support on the issue" (Otter 2011c).

Grant Money Rejected

Governor Otter's veto and executive order brought the issue of an insurance exchange to the forefront, though it would be another eight months before the legislature reconvened in January 2012. In the meantime, the executive branch tried to continue planning for the creation of a state-based exchange in case the legislature ultimately moved in that direction. However, in addition to being restricted by the Idaho Health Freedom Act of 2010, state agencies were not allowed to spend any money that the legislature had not explicitly appropriated, including grants it had received from the federal government.

A leader in the Department of Insurance explains that the timing of federal grants was complicated by the state's calendar. When the legislature is not in session, agencies are allowed to spend federal grant money if they have the governor's approval. When the legislature is back in session, it can refuse to appropriate this money going forward. The agency has to pay for it from its own budget if it wants to continue these activities (Interview June 2011). State agencies needed approval during the 2011 session in order to spend the $1 million exchange planning grant received the previous fall, as well as a $1 million grant to reform insurance rate review. An advisor to Governor Otter describes the careful way in which this request was framed to the legislature: "We explained why we wanted the money for planning, not really for implementation" (Interview June 2011).

The appropriations bill passed the Senate 20–15, but was not even voted on in the House (Idaho Senate Bill [SB] 1158 2011). Opponents argued that the money was "bait" and the state would be trapped into implementing the ACA if it accepted federal grants (Murphy 2011). Instead, the legislature appropriated $500,000 to support planning activities for the exchange and rate review. Supporters of an exchange were frustrated that not only would they only have a quarter of the money had they been allowed to spend the federal grants, but it would now come out of the state's budget instead of from federal grants (Interviews 2013–2014).

This episode was also an important moment for people who would play a key role in the final debate over an exchange. First, Wayne Hoffman of the IFF was largely given credit for making conservatives aware of the opportunity to resist Obamacare by blocking the appropriation of grant money, and then convincing them to take this step. This success was seen as another example of Hoffman's growing influence in state politics and strengthened his stature going into subsequent sessions (Interviews 2011–2013).

Second, the failure to pass the Department of Insurance budget was seen as a major blow to Director Bill Deal. One member of the House explains, "After the 2011 session, Deal continued to be an important contact with the Center for Consumer Information and Insurance Oversight (CCIIO), but took a backseat to the governor's office and the business community as far as driving this bill. I think that he didn't want to have his history be a determining factor" (Interview December 2011). Deal had served in the House for more than twenty-five years, having left the House after a failed bid to become speaker during the 2007 session. As a result, he had a complicated history with some of the people whose support he needed to create an exchange. As one legislator describes, “He was then rapidly moved from the House and was made the director of the Department of Insurance. This kind of protected him because House leaders Denney and Moyle would have had him sit on the back bench and just kind of play with him” (Interview December 2011).

With limited money and political support, there was little state bureaucrats could do to prepare for the creation of an exchange throughout 2011. They attempted to keep up with the federal timeline as much as possible, but largely shifted their focus to getting ready for the 2012 session. One Department of Insurance official explained, “We need legislation in place in the 2012 session . . . in order to meet the January 2013 deadline. Our goal is to have legislation out there in January 2012” so that the House and Senate can move quickly to consider their bill once in session (Interview June 2011).

NOVEMBER 2011—JUNE 2012

Three important events took place in Idaho during the period between when the US Supreme Court announced in November 2011 that it would hear the ACA case and when it ruled in June 2012: (1) the 2012 legislative session, (2) the development of a coalition of interest groups supporting state control of an exchange, and (3) the primary elections held on May 15. The last two significantly altered the political landscape for the 2013 session in which to create an exchange legislation would pass.

2012 Session

Many supporters of a state-based exchange were optimistic in the weeks leading up to the 2012 session that enabling legislation could pass. In the words of one House Democrat:

> My guess is there will be two bills we’ll have to deal with this year. One will be to do the statutory changes necessary for the exchange to exist. The other is an appropriations bill. Both of those will give opportunity for the nullifiers to rant and rave, carry flags, and throw bombs, and that kind of stuff. My feeling now is that there is enough understanding about what a state exchange versus a federal

> exchange means to businesses in the state of Idaho that they both might pass, actually. (Interview December 2011)

However, no exchange bills were even introduced during the 2012 session, let alone passed. Governor Otter told legislators he supported the concept of a state-run exchange, but he did little to push them to pass legislation. Wayne Hoffman of the IFF takes credit for this, saying, "A lot of that was our doing, putting the political pieces in place to stop the governor from being able to wrap his arms around that politically" (Interview April 2013). Others agree that the IFF played an important role, but cite House Speaker Lawerence Denney as the most important obstacle.

Speaker Denney strongly opposed all aspects of the ACA, including the creation of a state-based insurance exchange. He worked behind the scenes to ensure that if a bill was introduced it would not receive a hearing in committee. Interest group leaders closely watched to see if Representative Janice McGeachin, Chair of the House Health and Welfare Committee, would follow Speaker Denney or if she would let an exchange bill move forward. Shortly before the start of the session, she announced on an Idaho Falls radio show that she was against an exchange and would not allow legislation to proceed if anything came to her committee (Interviews 2012–2013).

Supporters of an exchange pressed Speaker Denney to at least allow the bill to come up for a vote. A lobbyist for one of the state's insurance companies believes that Denney was nervous that an exchange bill would probably pass if he gave it a hearing. Supporters of an exchange felt they had enough votes for a bill to pass the Senate and that they were close in the House. This person explains a series of frustrating encounters:

> I have never beaten my head against a wall so many times, because I would go see Lawerence Denney because he would say, "if you can do this, come back and talk and we'll see about giving it a hearing." I would then go do that and then he would move the goal post. He asked us to assure him that the majority of Republicans in the house would vote for it. We went out and we did that. We went back to him again and again and nothing. He strung it out. He knew exactly what he was doing. He kept stringing it out and stringing it out until there was no time left. Nothing happened. (Interview May 2013)

An advisor to Governor Otter explains that it would have been futile to push against House leadership over an exchange, and that trying to do so would be detrimental to the rest of his legislative agenda (Interview May 2013). There was little that supporters of an exchange could do to overcome opposition by Speaker Denney and Representative McGeachin without a strong commitment from Governor Otter. Even if they had succeeded in getting a hearing, it is unclear that enough Republicans would have joined the Democrats to pass a bill. Many hoped that the issue would go away as a result of the upcoming Supreme Court ruling and the upcoming presidential election (Interviews 2012–2013). Against these odds, legislation was never introduced.

Industry Coalition Develops

Interest groups decided to take a two-year approach to winning support for a state-based exchange when they realized legislation was not going to pass in 2012. Their strategy for the end of the 2012 session in March was to plant seeds and strengthen their coalition for next year's session (Interviews 2013). Two of Idaho's most powerful interest groups played a central role in this process: the Idaho Association of Commerce and Industry (IACI) and the Boise Metro Chamber of Commerce. Both organizations are influential because they represent a large number of Idaho's businesses, including groups with the greatest interest in an exchange such as healthcare providers and small business owners.

By 2012, both IACI and the Boise Metro Chamber had gone through a comprehensive internal process and determined that there was strong consensus in favor of a state-run exchange. Someone involved in IACI's process noted, "We don't have the ability in a small state like Idaho to call someone up in DC and resolve a problem promptly. We do have that opportunity in the state of Idaho. If we have a problem we can call the Department of Insurance and get a resolution in a hurry." This person adds, "Our view was that if we're going to do this, we're better off at least having the state have some level of control in the process" (Interview May 2013).

Leaders from these groups were frustrated by the arguments made by conservative organizations they often align with. As one person from the Boise Metro Chamber commented:

> To be frank, I was highly disappointed in the Cato Institute and those folks . . .. From a business perspective we have to do this regardless. They said that one way to get around this is to de-certify the licensing of all of our insurance companies in Idaho. That is a joke. The other way is to resist paying your taxes. That's

> a joke too. If you want to stay in business, the IRS doesn't give a damn what you're doing from that perspective; if you're not paying your taxes you'll get shut down. They were offering nothing except settling on a philosophical argument. We don't have that option; we have to conform. (Interview May 2013)

Not every interest group was in favor of a state-run exchange. One of the most prominent opponents was the Idaho Farm Bureau (IFB). Representing 64,000 Idahoan families in the agricultural industry, the Farm Bureau was one of the only groups to go on record in 2010 supporting the Idaho Health Freedom and in 2011 supporting the nullification bills. One of the organization's leaders acknowledges the tension over maintaining state control, saying, "I think it seems strange to people why we took this position. Generally, we are all in favor of the government most local doing the job. If the county can do it, then the county should do it. We don't want the federal government involved. It seems a little counter-intuitive that we'd be taking that position" (Interview May 2013). The organization's position was decided at the 2011 Annual Convention held in Coeur D'Alene. Republican Senators Russ Fulcher (against) and Dean Cameron (for) were invited to debate the pros and cons of a state-run insurance exchange, following which IFB members discussed the issue extensively and decided to "resist Obamacare in every possible way," including the exchange (Interview May 2013). The bottom-up nature of this process may have contributed to the Farm Bureau taking a different position than other industry groups that tended to have a more top-down decision-making process.

The interest group dynamic in Idaho was largely established by the time the Supreme Court ruled on June 28, 2012. Most of the traditionally powerful groups were in favor of an exchange. On the other side were a handful of industry opponents, such as the Idaho Farm Bureau, and ideology-driven groups such as the Tea Party and the IFF.

2012 Republican Primaries

The other major turning point during this period was the Republican Party primary elections held on May 15. Three factors made this election unique and consequential for the exchange debate. First, the caucus for the presidential campaign had already been held two months earlier. With the next gubernatorial election not until 2014, there was little on the ballot besides state legislative races. Turnout was not high. Second, this was the first election held since redistricting, which placed a number of incumbents against each other, leading many to retire. Third, this was the first time the state had a closed primary. There was an open ballot in the past, though Republicans accused Democrats of crossing over and voting for weak candidates (Wright 2012). More than one-third of Idaho's residents identify themselves as independents who could no longer vote in the Republican primary, meaning that the contests were likely dominated by the very most conservative people in the state (Russell 2012a).

These conditions created a perfect storm for infighting within the Republican Party that had important consequences for the debate over an exchange. House Speaker Lawerence Denney and House Majority Mike Moyle worked in an unprecedented way to strengthen control over their caucus. They funneled money from the House leadership political action committee (PAC)—the Victory Fund PAC—to a separate PAC targeting a handful of incumbent Republicans. One of the people targeted was another member of the House leadership team, Representative Ken Roberts. Moyle said Roberts had lied to him and threatened to defeat him. "My goal is to make Ken's life miserable because he's making my life miserable" (Russell 2012b). Roberts says this was not true, calling Denney's and Moyle's actions "disingenuous and highly disappointing" (Russell 2012c). Ironically, Roberts's position as a member of the House Leadership meant that he was treasurer of the Victory Fund that was being used to try to defeat him.

Denney and Moyle also targeted Republican Senator Dean Cameron, the cochair of the powerful Joint Finance and Appropriations Committee (JFAC) and a strong supporter of a state-run exchange. However, he and Roberts both survived their primary challenges. In fact, none of the candidates targeted by Denney and Moyle were defeated. Their unsuccessful attempts at unseating incumbent members of their caucus severely weakened their leadership in the House going into the 2013 legislative session.

According to Tea Party leaders, another narrative of the 2012 primaries was that insurers and other interest groups bought the election by spending large amounts of money to support advocates of a state-based exchange (Interviews 2012–2013). One Tea Party leader argued, "Our lawmakers are not rich. When you push around a couple hundred bucks in front of their noses and say 'let's going fishing,' or 'let's go to dinner,'—loyalty is easily and cheaply bought. 1042 and 248 are examples of exactly how cheap"[2] (Interview May 2013). There is limited evidence that this was the case. In fact, the Idaho Farm Bureau was the largest spender in races for the House, the chamber seen as most important for determining the outcome of the exchange debate. Blue Cross of Idaho was the fifteenth-largest spender at an amount one-third of the Idaho Farm Bureau's. Select Health was seventeenth and the Idaho Hospital Association was nineteenth. There was a very similar dynamic in Senate races (National Institute on Money in State Politics 2012).

One piece of evidence supporting the claim by Tea Party leaders is that IACI, a strong supporter of the exchange, was the third-largest spender during this election cycle in terms of independent expenditures. They spent a total of $89,613—quite a bit of money for Idaho politics—independently supporting candidates across the state, in addition to contributions made directly to each campaign. Yet, this was approximately the same amount as IACI had spent in the previous election cycle, before exchanges were on the legislative agenda (National Institute on Money in State Politics 2012), suggesting that this was not unusual or tied to any particular issue.

JULY 2012—OCTOBER 2013

It was unclear at the time what the primary election results would mean for the prospects of a state-run insurance exchange. Legislation had little chance of advancing as long as Lawerence Denney was Speaker. However, in the wake of the contentious primary season, there was talk that someone might challenge him for the speakership. The Supreme Court's decision in June and the national election results in November meant that Obamacare was still very much alive as legislators reconvened for the 2013 session. Infighting within the Republican Party would culminate in March 2013 with the passage of HB 248, creating an insurance exchange.

2013 Organizational Session

Reelected and newly elected legislators meet every other December to select their leaders for the next two years. The organizational session is often a formality in which the previous officers are reelected. Occasionally there are heated contests to fill open positions, but it is rare for a current leader to be challenged by a member of his or her party. As legislators met in December 2012 to prepare for the 2013 session starting a few weeks later, many Republicans were upset with Speaker Denney and House Majority Moyle for trying to defeat incumbents in the previous primary. Their approach to legislating was also unpopular, with members of their caucus describing them as vindictive, closed, and holding on to grudges (Interviews 2013). Representative Scott Bedke of Oakley saw an opening and decided to make a run at the Speakership.

Bedke conducted a highly personalized campaign to win enough support within the Republican caucus. Redistricting and retirements in 2012 meant that more than a third of the legislature would be new in 2013. As Denney and Moyle were making enemies of Republican incumbents throughout the 2012 campaign season, Bedke focused on helping Republicans running for open seats. Many of these Republican freshmen explain that he personally drove out to their remote corner of the state to give his support (Interviews 2013). Bedke contributed between $200 and $1,250 to the campaigns of all but one of the twenty-three newly elected House Republicans (National Institute on Money in State Politics 2012). This was not enough money to swing an election for most candidates, but it was a symbol of involvement and support. Denney's Victory Fund PAC contributed to all but five of the newly elected House Republicans, meaning that Bedke had contributed to four more new legislators than had Denney. The vote for speaker was a closed ballot, but many interviewed say it was close enough that four people may have made the difference (Interviews 2013).

Interest groups had a lot at stake in the speaker's race, though none got involved publicly. A leader of a business organization compared lobbying about the leadership race to "playing with fire" (Interview May 2013). Another industry representative explained, "There is one sacred area that lobbyists will not engage in, and that is the politics of leadership" (Interview May 2013). The risk of backing the wrong candidate and being outcast by the new leadership was too great. In other words, the most important moment in the 2013 legislative session had no direct engagement from interest groups.

This was one of the most important turning points in the debate over an exchange even though it had nothing directly to do with the politics of health reform. Scott Bedke's election as speaker meant that the idea of creating a state-run insurance exchange might be allowed to progress. Speaker Bedke did not initially indicate whether he would support an exchange, but made it clear he would allow bills to be introduced, hearings to be held, and votes to be called on controversial issues. A member of the House explained, "There was a different leadership style and culture, leading to a different feel in the House" (Interview May 2013).

Speaker Bedke ultimately decided to support an exchange. A Republican senator who supported an exchange said, "It changed the whole dynamic. If [an exchange] was going to get hung up, it would probably be in the House, which is where the opposition to that type of thing had been the strongest in the past" (Interview May 2013). Another Republican senator describes Speaker Bedke's evolution on the exchange:

> At least he wanted to give the bill an opportunity to be heard. In fact, to speaker Bedke's credit, he spent literally hours learning about the pros and cons, and learning about the issues. He became very knowledgeable. With that knowledge, he decided that the decision to have a state-based exchange was preferable compared to the federal exchange. He became a proponent. (Interview May 2013)

Bedke's support was particularly consequential because he had the power to decide which committee an exchange bill would be sent to, who chaired the committee, and which members sat on the committee. Representative Janice McGeachin had retired the previous year, meaning that the position of chair of the House Health and Welfare Committee was open. Bedke appointed Fred Wood, a physician who was one of the people representing the legislature on Governor Otter's exchange task force and who was a big proponent of Idaho retaining control. Tea Party leaders and even supporters of an exchange suggest that it appears Bedke stacked the Health and Welfare Committee to pass exchange legislative, noting that along with the Democrats, he already had enough votes to get the bill out of committee before a bill was even introduced (Interviews 2013). As supporters of an exchange would soon find out, this did not ensure that a bill would ultimately make it out of the House and be signed into law.

But it did help that many of the people now in key decision-making positions worked in the healthcare industry. Fred Wood is a physician and medical director at the Cassia Regional Medical Center. House Minority Leader John Rusche is a retired physician who worked for many years in the health insurance industry. Five members of the legislature are insurance brokers, including Senator Dean Cameron, cochair of the powerful Joint Finance and Appropriations Committee; Senator John Goedde, chair of the Senate Education Committee; and Representative Gary Collins, chair of the House Revenue and Taxation Committee. Each of these people became sources of information for the rest of the legislature on issues dealing with health insurance and became an important leader on the exchange debate. Fred Wood's leadership was particularly important for passage in the House, the chamber where legislation was most likely to suffer defeat.

Governor Otter Deliberates

Governor Otter was free to support a state-based exchange now that Lawerence Denney was no longer blocking legislation. The only reason this was still an option for the state in December 2012 was because the Department of Health and Human Serices (HHS) had pushed the previous deadline of November 16 back a month. Senate leadership met with Governor Otter in mid-November, shortly after the deadline extension, but before Scott Bedke had become the new speaker. They were concerned with the possibility the governor would try to create an exchange on his own in the absence of legislation. Senate leaders saw this as a separation of powers issue even more important than an exchange, saying, "We wanted to make sure we had a pattern in place that says the legislature, as hard as it is to wrestle with these issues, should have to" (Interview April 2013). They consulted with a private law firm to explore their options in case the governor acted on his own. One person summarized the November meeting saying, "He made us a—I don't know if the word is a promise—but I certainly left that meeting confident that he was not going to issue an executive order to make a decision without including us" (Interview May 2013).

Governor Otter went through a surprisingly involved deliberation over the exchange, considering that he had supported the concept the year before. In December, he told the leadership teams from both chambers that he had not yet decided what to do. Otter read from a recent press release by Governor Chris Christie explaining why he had vetoed legislation in New Jersey. Legislative leaders told him that Otter would not advance legislation if he was not going to support it. One person in the room explains, "I honestly left that meeting thinking that he's not going to do this" (Interview April 2013).

Another meeting was scheduled for the following week, just days before the new HHS deadline to declare a state's intention to create an exchange. All four members of the Senate leadership were in attendance, but Speaker Bedke was the only leader from the House. Governor Otter announced that he was going to support a state-based exchange. Senator Majority Leader Bart Davis referred to this moment during the Senate debate, quoting Governor Otter as saying that this was the second-hardest decision he has made in public office, only behind his vote in Congress to oppose the Patriot Act (ID Senate Debate, February 21, 2013).

Governor Otter was under pressure from business interests supporting an exchange and far right Republicans who were opposed. An advisor explains that he went to a Republican Governor's Association meeting around this time where others hoped for a united front against Obamacare. "He knew how everyone was feeling, that if we all don't do it, the whole thing would fall apart" (Interview May 2013). This argument had persuaded Governor Phil Bryant to resist an exchange in Mississippi, but did not sway Governor Otter.

Interest group leaders praised the governor for his support. A prominent insurance agent said, "Otter put forth an enormous amount of courage, saying I know my party is against this and thinks I'm stupid, but I have to think about what's best for the state of Idaho. My opinion from talking to Otter, his staff, the Department of Insurance, the people I've talked to over the last two years, I really think he came down with the decision that the businesses and people he talked to didn't think he had a choice" (Interview May 2013). Another industry leader added, "By that time, the Supreme Court had ruled and Romney had lost. So the grand scenario for Republicans was not going to take place. Otter said we may not like it, but it's the law of the law of the land" (Interview My 2013).

Having decided to support an exchange, Governor Otter now faced a number of other challenges, including how to meet the Obama administration's December deadline while the legislature was out of session until January, how strongly to push the legislature, and what tactics to employ. This moment was widely seen as a huge test of leadership for Governor Otter (Russell 2013a). The first challenge was easily overcome, as leaders at HHS were more than happy to cooperate with a Republican governor trying to create an exchange in a solidly red state. An advisor to Governor Otter explained, "It's not that we gained a seat at the table, at this point we feel like we created the table. We really have gotten a lot of concessions from them and they really do want us to succeed. There are other states that don't have that" (Interview May 2013). In fact, this advisor explains that other Republican governors who were publicly opposing Obamacare were privately asking Otter to advocate to HHS on their behalf, observing that he had a relationship they did not (Interview May 2013).

Governor Otter's decision in December 2012 to fully support an Idaho-run exchange raised the stakes for the debate. It was no longer just a question of implementing a component of Obamacare, but a test of leadership for the "Gentleman on the second floor" (the phrase many legislators used during floor debates when speaking about the governor, referencing the location of his office one floor below the House and Senate chambers). Governor Otter decided to put the full weight of his office behind a state-based exchange. He spoke strongly in favor of an exchange during his state of the state speech on the first day of the session in January 2013 (Otter 2013). The governor's staff took the lead in coordinating lobbying groups in favor of an exchange, as well as drafting legislation. David Hensley and Tammy Perkins, Governor Otter's Chief of Staff and health policy advisor, held regular breakfast and lunch meetings with legislators throughout the session to answer questions about an exchange.

Governor Otter even had Hensley introduce exchange legislation and testify in committee hearings in the House and Senate as a "governor's bill." This is a simple power not available to governors in every state. A bill in the Idaho legislature needs a floor sponsor from the House and Senate in order to be considered by the full body of each chamber, but can be introduced in committee by someone else. The vast majority of bills are carried in committee by the same person who becomes the floor sponsor. In 2013, there were 345 bills introduced in the House and 200 introduced in the Senate.[3] The only time David Hensley introduced a bill was for the insurance exchange.[4] Having his chief of staff introduce the legislation instead sent a powerful message to legislators that this was a high priority for Governor Otter.

Stakeholders on both sides of the debate stressed the importance of Governor Otter's support. One opponent said, "The fact that the governor supported an exchange in Idaho was key. If he hadn't, the idea would have been dead on arrival" (Interview April 2013). Others noted that the amount of time dedicated to this issue by Hensley and Perkins indicated how important an issue this was for Governor Otter (Interviews 2013). An industry leader praised Hensley, saying, "He was brilliant at calmly explaining the merits of an exchange. He had an outstanding demeanor . . .. I thought he did a masterful job" (Interview may 2013). Tea Party leaders were angry, calling him a traitor (Interviews 2013).

SB 1042 Introduced

An early strategic decision legislative leaders had to make was which chamber should consider the bill first. The legislative process in some states resembles that of Congress, in which chambers work on similar legislation in parallel and resolve differences through a conference committee. By contrast, legislation in Idaho is typically considered one chamber at a time. In other words, the Senate does not consider a bill until after it has been approved by the House, and vice versa.

Many Senators strongly preferred that the process begin in the House, since it was likely to be the more difficult chamber. They did not want to have to take a tough vote if they did not have to (Interviews 2013). Much to their frustration, Senate Pro Tempore Brent Hill agreed to start the process in the Senate, hoping that a solid victory there would generate momentum going into the House debate. Also, turnover in the House was particularly high, with thirty of the seventy representatives being brand new. As one legislative leader explained, "This was a very hot and emotional issue. Starting in the Senate gave [new legislators] more time for the learning curve" (Interview May 2013).

Senate Bill 1042 was introduced on January 30 in the Senate Commerce and Human Resources Committee, the Senate committee that typically handles insurance legislation. Senators note that unlike in the House, where the speaker has significant discretion over committee assignments, senators get to select their committees according to seniority. As a result, it was not possible for Senate leaders to stack the committee in favor of an exchange. However, it did help that two members of the committee, Senators Dean Cameron and John Goedde are both insurance agents during the rest of the year when the legislature is not in session. A fellow senator on the committee explains, "They had the background information to answer the technical questions," and played a leadership role behind the scenes (Interview May 2013).

Committee chairman Senator John Tippets anticipated a large crowd and a heated debate at the bill's committee hearing on February 5. He would not be able to accommodate everyone that came to testify, but wanted to make sure everyone felt heard. He gave each person three minutes to speak. The only exceptions were the ten minutes to Governor Otter's chief of staff and Wayne Hoffman, head of the IFF, who was considered the de facto leader of opposing an exchange.

The IFF is not officially affiliated with the Tea Party but played an important role in filling what could be considered a leadership void. The decentralized nature of the Tea Party movement, combined with the size and sparseness of the state, meant that it was difficult for each of the disparate groups to organize and clearly articulate a message. Hoffman described the IFF as "ammo suppliers" for the Tea Party through its website The Idaho Reporter, which is regularly updated with summaries and YouTube videos about state government (Idaho Reporter 2014). Hoffman explained, "We provide ammunition. We provide information. We provide details and research. It's available to the general public of course, but one of the biggest consumers of this information are people in the Tea Party who believe in limited government as we do" (Interview April 2013). Armed with this information and educated on the legislative process, Tea Party groups turned out in large numbers for the February 5 committee hearing.

After Hensley and Hoffman spoke, testimony alternated between supporters and opponents, and so it was not obvious from testimony alone which side had a greater presence. Supporters tended to be from industry, praising the advantages of local control. Opponents tended to be private citizens, warning about a government takeover of healthcare. One person testified that by supporting an exchange, the governor was accepting full ownership of the ACA, and that in Idaho the law would now be known as "Ottercare" (Russell 2013b).

At the conclusion of the meeting, Senator Tippets thanked everyone for holding a civil debate. He explained that the meeting would continue two days later so more people would have an opportunity to speak. On February 7, the legislative auditorium was once again packed. This time, a large number of audience members wore bright pink pieces of duct tape on their lapels. A senator on the committee explains, "Our rules are clear that people are not allowed to bring signs or wear pins that have a message, but they wanted the committee to know that most people in attendance were opposed to an exchange, and this was a creative way of doing this" (Interview May 2013). Despite a strong showing and aggressive testimony by the Tea Party, the committee passed SB 1042 by a vote of 8–1 (Russell 2013c). The only no vote came from a Democrat who supported the concept of an exchange but wanted more legislative oversight. Governor Otter put out a statement saying that he was proud of Senate Republicans for voting unanimously in favor of state control of the exchange (Russell 2013d).

A few days later, SB 1042 appeared on the Senate docket for a floor debate and vote. Without explanation, the debate was pushed back. As the bill came up for a debate again, the same thing happened. After nearly a week of delays it was reported that a group of sixteen House freshmen were about to introduce their own exchange bill (Popkey 2013). The typical legislative process in Idaho was now being turned on its head.

The Freshmen 16

As SB 1042 made its way through the Senate, some House Republicans expressed frustration over the choice they would soon need to make. They did not like Obamacare, but wanted state control of the exchange, including strong legislative oversight, and SB 1042 gave control of Idaho's exchange to an independent board of directors that did not include any legislators or people appointed by the legislature (Idaho Senate Bill [SB] 1042 2013). One freshman Republican explains, "I felt like a fish out of water flopping all around, because one second I'm going, ya, this part makes sense. Maybe we'll do this and not be complicit, but then I'd think 'no, I don't want this to happen,' and I was flip flopping all over the place. And it was not a very comfortable feeling" (Interview April 2013).

Representative Luke Malek had similar feelings and began having informal conversations with fellow freshmen Republicans. He sensed discontent from enough people that he organized a meeting in which options were discussed. This group of sixteen new legislators decided to write a trailer bill to the Senate bill, meaning that their bill could only become law if SB 1042 was also passed. Legislation was drafted the next morning, and they went to Speaker Bedke and Governor Otter that afternoon. They announced their plans at a press conference the following morning (Interviews 2013).

Members of the Freshmen 16 say the speaker and governor were very receptive because head counts made it clear that SB 1042 was not going to pass the House (Interviews 2013). These freshmen were a lifeline toward winning enough support. Not all Republicans were as receptive. House Republican Brent Crane called Luke Malek to the Capitol Building late one night. When Malek arrived, US Congressman and former state legislator Raul Labrador was there to confront him. Labrador reportedly made threats to try and convince him to back off on the exchange, but Malek was undeterred (Interviews 2013).

It is interesting that Luke Malek only organized freshmen, and not all House Republicans supporting an exchange. One member of the group of sixteen freshmen explains that none of the freshmen had been around for the previous fights over the Idaho Health Care Freedom Act and thus did not have the same entrenched positions as other legislators (Interview May 2013). Another notes, "The freshmen found ourselves in a unique position as the new girl at the dance and no one is asking us to dance. So we got together to watch each other's backs. The people we could trust the most were the people in our same shoes" (Interview December 2013).

Leaders on both sides of the debate over an exchange cite the press conference on February 13 by the House Freshmen as an important turning point. An official at the Department of Insurance says, "That group of 16 was a momentum changer without any question" (Interview May 2013). A leader at the Idaho Farm Bureau, one of the few industry groups opposed to an exchange, explains, "The odds were stacked up against us, but we felt we had a chance until the gang of 16. . . . That's what changed everything. Until that moment, we thought many of those freshmen were in play" to vote against an exchange (Interview May 2013).

Senate Passes SB 1042

It took a few days for Senate leaders to decide how to react to the freshmen. While SB 1042 had already passed the Senate Commerce and Human Resources Committee, it had not been voted on by the full body. It was determined that the Senate would try to pass SB 1042 and then consider the trailer bill if it passed the House. One Senate leader explained that House leaders appealed to the Senate, saying, "This is about trust; that you run the original bill over to us and we'll send you the trailer bill. Once you pass the trailer bill, then we'll take up the other one" (Interview April 2013).

The Senate began debating unusually early on February 21, with an announcement from leadership that, given the tensions around an exchange, there would be no time limit and that they would continue until everyone said everything they wanted to say (Russell 2013e). The prayer by the Senate Chaplain that morning asked that Senators be "inspired with good visions" and "guided through each quandary" (ID Senate Debate February 21, 2013). The marathon session went on for more than six hours. Unlike in Congressional debates, where statements are generally made before empty chambers as legislators come and go, the vast majority of Idaho's Senators remained for the entire debate.

The debate was passionate, but remarkably respectful. Before the meeting, Senate Pro Tempore Brent Hill told the caucus that he would be sitting in the chair presiding over the chamber and would not tolerate incivility (Interviews 2013). One opponent of an exchange who did not like the outcome expressed, "It was probably some of the greatest debate we have ever seen in recent memory of Idaho politics . . .. People entered the chamber as friends and left as friends" (Interview April 2013).

Arguments were either framed in terms of ideology or the benefits of local control. Insurance agents such as Senator Cameron and Senator Goedde argued that an exchange run by Idaho could keep user fees low and ensure that fewer insurance mandates would be included. Senator Hagerdorn used a unique analogy to explain why he supported an exchange even though he opposed Obamacare. "Our choice is a federal exchange or a state exchange. I can't ride this pig if it's a federal exchange. I can ride it with spurs on if it's a state exchange. I select the one that I have at least the ability to spur once in a while." An argument in favor of state control given by Senator Cameron and Senator Davis was that if the Obama administration is able to set up exchanges in most states, then they are just one push of a button away from establishing a single-payer system. Senator Fulcher disagreed, saying that complying with Obamacare to any degree put the state on a path toward a single-payer system. He used coded language referencing Mormon scripture, "In my heart and in my mind,[5] I know where this leads, and there is no turning back once we do it."

The rhetoric turned a bit more heated by the fourth hour. Senator Rice declared the ACA unconstitutional, regardless of the Supreme Court's ruling, saying, "John Roberts is a Supreme Court Justice and needs to act like it!" Senator Pearce appealed to the state's culture of independence and resistance, saying, "Liberty is the right to choose. Freedom is the result of a choice. . . . Come on folks, this is Idaho!" Senator McKenzie referenced a Russian author writing in a concentration camp during World War II. The author was quoted as saying, "We didn't love freedom enough" before then and, "we deserved what happened afterward." Senator McKenzie concluded, "I will not be complicit in the federal government taking control. This echoed a comment made on Twitter earlier by Senator Sheryl Nuxoll, who compared the role of insurance companies in an exchange to "the Jews boarding the trains to concentration camps" because she believed it made abortion more accessible (Russell 2013f).

At the end of the long debate, the Senate voted 23–12 to pass SB 1042. Senators on both sides say that no one changed their minds as a result of the debate, with the final vote exactly as they had predicted at the outset. However, it was not clear what would happen next, including whether the House would pass both SB 1042 and the trailer bill, and whether the Senate would then pass the trailer bill.

HB 248 Introduced in the House

A hearing on the House freshmen's trailer bill, HB 179 (Idaho House Bill [HB] 179), was originally scheduled for February 22, the day after the Senate debate and vote. Without public explanation, the bill was then removed from the agenda of the House Health and Welfare Committee. There were concerns from House members about the agreement between the leaders of the two chambers over the improvised process. The trailer bill technically could not be passed until after the bill it trailed had passed. In other words, the House would first have to approve SB 1042 before considering the trailer bill, and then would have to rely on the Senate to win enough votes to pass the trailer bill. This left House freshmen vulnerable to the possibility that the bill passed by the Senate would become law while the changes they wanted would not. The solution was for an entirely new bill to be drafted, incorporating elements from the governor's bill as well as the increased legislative oversight demanded by the sixteen House freshmen. Senate leaders agreed to this plan, but were frustrated that it meant they would have to debate exchange legislation once again (Interviews 2013).

Interest groups on both sides were mobilized in high gear by the time HB 248 was introduced in the House on March 4. In addition to coordinating large groups to show up at the legislative hearings, as when they wore pink duct tape to the Senate committee hearing, Tea Party leaders attacked legislators in their home districts. The local Republican Party organization in some counties held votes of no confidence for their freshmen House members who supported an exchange. One interest group leader describes these as "huge, awful meetings that were shouting matches in which the police was almost called they were so unruly. They absolutely demeaned these legislators in front of all these people. . . . It's pretty ugly at the precinct level" (Interview May 2013).

Though loud and aggressive, it was unclear how representative these opponents were of the rest of Idahoans. A Republican legislative leader tried to put the Tea Party opposition in perspective, comparing it to the public outcry over a bill that would have removed the sales tax exemption for Girl Scout cookies. "If you take the amount of email I received in a given week on the girl scouts sales tax exemption, and compare it to the total number of emails I received the whole year on the state-based exchange, the girls scout cookies sales tax exemption was substantially more. What you have is a very loud, obnoxious, but small group of opponents."

On the other side, the industry coalition coordinated by Governor Otter's office, known as the Idaho Health Exchange Alliance, now included more than four hundred businesses. The Idaho Association of Health Plans provided money for the Alliance to hire a private public relations firm to do grassroots work. The Alliance ran radio ads with Governor Otter advocating for state control of the exchange. A website called KeepitinIdaho.com was developed to showcase the strength of the coalition and included a long list of businesses and individuals supporting an exchange.

An advisor to Governor Otter explains, "All the legislators were hearing from the far right; they were inundated from the far right. If you're only hearing from the far right you wonder where everyone else is and figure no one cares. So the goal of the Alliance was to get other people involved and get them to speak up" (Interview May 2013). Describing the effects of the industry coalition on the debate, one legislative leader says, "I think it was huge. It gave people courage. I'm not saying they wouldn't have done it anyway, but it certainly helped buoy up our courage." One House leader estimated, "In the 2013 session, more than half, maybe three-fourths of the full-time lobbyists were working on this issue—mostly in favor" (Interview May 2013). Many said the IACI and Chamber Alliance were the two most important industry allies. "When you have got your business groups as a whole supporting this, that helps. We tout ourselves as a pro-business state. How do you vote against something that the majority of your businesses support?" (Interview May 2013).

Lobbying for the exchange in Idaho actually began well before the start of the 2013 session. Many industry groups used their PACs to get involved in elections. One insurance industry lobbyist said they spent much of the summer of 2012 meeting as many of the Republicans campaigning for open seats as possible. This person adds, "It paid off tremendously for me as most of them were elected and I knew them by the time the session started" (Interview May 2013).

Opponents accuse the insurance industry of buying the exchange through their contributions in the previous election. However, analysis of campaign finance data reveals there is no clear pattern between the money legislators received in 2012 and how they voted on HB 248 in 2013 (National Institute on Money in State Politics 2012). Even so, the lobbyist for one insurance company said, "We let it be known to legislators that the exchange was our number one issue." Speaking of the House freshmen who voted for an exchange, this person added, "I have told them they have my undying loyalty and support for whatever it is they need for their campaign" (Interview May 2013). This person clarified that there was not an explicit quid pro quo relationship in which votes were bought, but an acknowledgment that they were willing to help legislators who were being threatened from the right as a result of their exchange vote. House members describe these interactions in similarly soft terms, but also point out that insurance companies gave them campaign donations shortly after the legislative session (Interviews 2013).

On Thursday March 7, interest groups on both sides packed the legislative auditorium—which had been named after Abraham Lincoln since the Senate Commerce and Human Resources Committee held its hearing a month earlier. The hearing on HB 248 began at 7 a.m. to give as much time for testimony as possible. Governor Otter's chief of staff introduced the bill once again, followed by opposing arguments from IFF leader Wayne Hoffman. Twelve people testified in favor of HB 248, including many of the leaders of the industry coalition. Twenty-six people testified against the law, including at least fifteen who identified themselves as member of the Tea Party or had an online presence as a member of the Tea Party. Two were members of antiabortion groups, and two were leaders in their county Republican Party organizations. These were very large numbers for an Idaho legislative committee. By comparison, a combined total of thirteen people testified about the sixteen pieces of legislation considered at the previous five meetings of the House Health and Welfare Committee (Idaho House Health and Welfare 2013).

The main argument put forward by Tea Party leaders was that HB 248 presented a false choice. In the words of one person who spoke against the bill, "We've only got two choices, a state-run or a federally run exchange. Which do you want? That's a lie. The third, fourth, and fifth choice is nullification. There's do nothing and let the 2010 Idaho Health Freedom Act prevail (Interview May 2013). Another opponent told legislators that

REAL ID was an example of an instance in which the federal government backed off of requirements because so many states refused to comply (Interview May 2013). Despite such heated arguments, the committee passed HB 248 on a voice vote. Only Representative VanderWoude asked that his opposition be included in the record (Idaho House Health and Welfare Committee 2013).

HB 248 Passes House and Senate

Interest groups lobbied aggressively in the week between the House Health and Welfare Committee hearing on March 7 and the debate on the House floor on March 13. Anticipating that the outcome of the Senate vote on HB 248 would be similar to the previous vote on SB 1042, opponents saw this as their last best chance to beat an exchange. The tone of the House debate was mostly civil, though occasionally heated. Most House members remained in the chamber for the duration of the seven-hour debate. The House gallery was filled with opponents of an exchange, including the state Republican Party Chairman, who reportedly led applause when opponents spoke. One legislator believed, "This was very inappropriate; very out of line; very unprofessional. He later did send an email to all the legislators, at least the Republicans, sort of apologizing. It was more of an 'If I wasn't supposed to do that, I'm sorry,' but he's not really admitting that he did anything wrong" (Interview April 2013).

The split within the Republican caucus meant the House was effectively divided into three factions, Republicans who supported an exchange, Republicans who opposed an exchange, and Democrats. This put the Democratic caucus in the unusual position of being the deciding votes even though they only had thirteen seats. An interest group leader explains that although most people expected the Democrats to support a state-based exchange, it was not a foregone conclusion. "We didn't know until the day before what they were going to do" (Interview May 2013). Some Democrats wanted to use the situation as leverage, refusing to vote for the Republican exchange bill unless their education bills were supported in return. House Minority Leader John Rusche reportedly talked his caucus out of using the exchange debate this way because the two issues were unrelated and unlinked in people's minds. They also did not want to risk being the reason a state exchange was not created. As one member of the caucus explains, "very few were actually willing to shoot the hostage" (Interview September 2013).

Interest group leaders and Republican supporters of an exchange praise the approach taken by Representative Rusche and the Democrats.

One House Republican said, "They did not say one word throughout the whole debate. They were very wise in understanding that this was a party-specific argument. They knew where they were and that they wouldn't be changing minds" (Interview May 2013). In fact, they knew that they might make it harder for Republicans to support an exchange if the issue was closely identified with Democrats rather than Governor Otter and other Republicans (Interviews 2013).

When the roll call was finally taken, HB 248 passed 41–29 (Idaho House of Representatives 2013). Two of the freshmen sixteen ended up voting no, meaning that there were ultimately more Republicans (29) voting against the bill than voting for it (28). Democrats made up the difference, with all thirteen voting in favor.

The Senate then moved quickly on SB 248 so it could be passed by the end of the session less than three weeks away. Senator Tippets began the hearing on March 19 by referencing criticism that he had erred by not disclosing a conflict of interest as a member of IACI's board of directors. He acknowledged that IACI is a primary supporter of an exchange, but explained his belief that there was no conflict of interest and that the attorney general's office agreed there was no conflict (Idaho Senate Commerce and Human Resources Committee 2013).

Once again, David Hensley introduced the bill on behalf of the governor and Wayne Hoffman spoke first for the opponents. Many of the same people that testified to the Senate on SB 1042 and to the House on HB 248 testified again. Tea Party leader Chad Inman warned, "Lies will come out and will continue to be told." He added that he does not blame the committee "because they are under a lot of pressure from lobbyists and the governor" (Idaho Senate Commerce and Human Resources Committee 2013).

Senator Sheryl Nuxoll, most known in this debate for comparing an exchange to the holocaust, took the unusual step of testifying against a bill before a committee in the other chamber. She cited her Catholic faith and warned that an exchange would increase access to emergency contraception that was on par with abortion. She was followed by Christine Tiddens of the Catholic Charities of Idaho, who disagreed, saying that the Diocese of Idaho supported creating an exchange in general and HB 248 in particular. The committee passed HB 248 by a vote of 8–1. The only no vote once again came from Democrat Brandon Durst, even though this bill seemed to address the criticisms he had raised when voting against SB 1042 (Idaho Senate Commerce and Human Resources Committee 2013). Durst was the youngest member of the legislature at thirty-three years old. A Republican Senator describes Durst's opposition as obstinance rather than a principled or influential stand. "Nobody listens to him. He is irrelevant. He is not only irrelevant, he is irrelevant in his own caucus. . . . That is the single least impressive, if not the worst, freshmen year I have ever seen. . . . He wants to debate everything" (Interview April 2013).

The full Senate voted two days later to pass HB 248. The roll call was the exact same as for SB 1042, with twenty-three in favor and twelve opposed. Nobody expected a different outcome, but that hardly meant that the debate was a quick formality. The session started with Republican Senator Dean Mortimer objecting to the unanimous consent to waive the full reading of the bill, meaning that everyone sat and listened as the Senate's secretary took ten minutes to read the entire bill (Russell 2013g). The debate lasted more than three hours, with critics making many of the same attacks against the exchange and supporters giving many of the same defenses as during the previous debate.

The tone was once again passionate but respectful. Near the end of the debate, Senate Pro Tempore Brent Hill said, "Many will criticize your choice here today, either way you vote, because the choices we have stink. But the critics are wrong if they question what's in your heart, and I thank you for what I see in your hearts. I'm proud of you." Though the debate was once again remarkably civil and their preferences prevailed, legislators supporting an exchange privately described this as their most frustrating session and the most divided they had ever seen the legislature (Interviews 2013).

Governor Otter released a statement shortly after the vote, saying, "I appreciate the legislature's support enabling me to do what I believe is right for our citizens. Of course we share objections to Obamacare, but as responsible elected officials we are also committed to constructively working for the best possible outcomes for Idaho. I'm grateful for that collaboration" (Hill 2013). Governor Otter signed HB 248 into law one week later on March 28.

Post-Session

In the closing days of the 2013 session, House Minority Leader John Rusche introduced a bill to expand Medicaid. The idea was effectively dead on arrival, since Governor Otter indicated in his state of the state speech three months earlier that he would not support Medicaid expansion that year. Legislation was not likely to proceed without his support. Even if Otter had reversed, many Republican supporters of the exchange privately expressed that they were burnt out on discussing the Affordable Care Act and could not imagine sticking their necks out again. The exchange debate had dominated the session for so long that there was not time to consider Medicaid before sine die, or the end of the session. This left Idaho as the only state during the ACA's first full year of implementation (2014) to have chosen a state run exchange while rejecting the Medicaid expansion (Jones, Singer, and Ayanian 2014).

Governor Otter appointed nineteen people to the exchange's board of directors on April 10, just two weeks after HB 248 was signed into law. These appointments did not need immediate Senate confirmation, because they were made after the legislative session had concluded, if only by a matter of days. The board included a wide range of people, such as consumer advocates, providers, insurers, agents, and legislators. However, one of the consequences of having taken so long to decide to run its exchange is that Idaho's policymakers did not have enough time to develop the IT before open enrollment began in October 2013.

An agreement was struck with the federal government that the board of Idaho's exchange would retain some policymaking authority, but the state would rely on the federal website healthcare.gov for the first year. Opponents of an exchange cite this as evidence that they were right all along, that Idaho would not really have that much control over its exchange. The *Wall Street Journal* criticized Idaho for having fought so intensely for control only to give it back to the federal government (Dooren 2013). Wayne Hoffman says, "The whole thing would be laughable if it wasn't such a disgrace" (Interview October 2013). However, supporters were adamant that Idaho was not using a federal exchange but it should be considered a "supported state exchange" (Interview October 2013).

This intergovernmental dynamic created confusing situations for Idahoans during the first weeks of open enrollment in October 2013. One official describes that when the federal website did not work, consumers would phone the Idaho call center in Boise. The staff of ten people was not able to do much other than refer people to healthcare.gov and give them the phone number for the federal call center. When people then called the federal call center, they were told that Idaho was running its own exchange and so they should call the Idaho call center. If they did call back, it was to complain that one side was either uninformed or lying (Interview October 2013).

It is hard to find a state in which the Republican opposition to the ACA was stronger than in Idaho. It was the first state in the nation to pass legislation opposing the reform. It was one of the original states to join the lawsuits against the individual mandate and the Medicaid expansion. The legislature passed bills in 2011 declaring the ACA null and void within the state's borders. Even so, strong gubernatorial leadership, a strong interest group coalition, and legislative pockets of expertise helped Idaho became the only state led entirely by Republicans that chose to create an exchange.

CHAPTER 5

New Mexico

INTRODUCTION

New Mexico and Idaho were the last two states to decide to create a health insurance exchange.[1] Coincidentally, Governor Susana Martinez signed New Mexico's legislation on the same day as Governor Butch Otter signed Idaho's—March 28, 2013. Idaho's decision was surprising, given that it is one of the most conservative states in the country and the only state led entirely by Republicans to choose this path. The surprise in New Mexico was that it took this long and almost did not happen.

When the Affordable Care Act was signed into law in March 2010, the political climate in New Mexico seemed favorable to implementing reform. Barack Obama was popular, having won 57% of the vote in 2008 against John McCain of neighboring Arizona (New Mexico [NM] Secretary of State 2012, see Table 5.1). All five members of the state's congressional delegation were Democrats, and all but one voted for the ACA (United States Senate Vote #396 2010; United States House Roll Call #165 2010). Democrats had controlled both chambers of the legislature for more than two decades and held 64% of seats in each chamber (NCSL 2010b). Democrat Bill Richardson was in his fourth and final year of a second term as governor largely defined by advancing health reform. In fact, the state had already done similar versions of reforms included in the ACA, such as establishing a medical loss ratio of 85% and allowing children to stay on their parents plan until age twenty-five. Republicans had been trying for many years to create an insurance exchange for small businesses (Interviews 2013).

The first exchange bills were introduced in 2007 and 2008, largely at the urging of J. R. Damron, a radiologist from Santa Fe who was the Republican nominee for governor in 2006. He explains that he did not feel his party had a plan for healthcare. "After looking at the Massachusetts program and

Table 5.1. NEW MEXICO'S POLITICAL AND DEMOGRAPHIC CONTEXT

Political Environment

- 2012 presidential election: Barack Obama (53%)
- Governor
  - 2003–2010: Bill Richardson (D)
  - 2011–present: Susana Martinez (R)
  - Term limits: two terms of four years each
- New Mexico House of Representatives
  - 2011–2012: Democratic majority of four
  - 2013–2015: Democratic majority of eight
  - No term limits
- New Mexico Senate
  - 2011–2012: Democratic majority of twelve
  - 2013–2015: Democratic majority of seven
  - No term limits

Demographics & Health Status

- Total population: 2,048,000
- Distribution of Population by Federal Poverty Level
  - Under 100%: 27%
  - 100%–138%: 8%
  - 139%–399%: 36%
  - 400%: 30%
- Distribution of Health Insurance Coverage
  - Employer: 38%
  - Other private: 5%
  - Medicaid: 21%
  - Medicare: 15%
  - Uninsured: 21%

Health Reform

- Did not join lawsuit against the ACA
- State-based exchange, relying on national website for first year
- Expanding Medicaid

what the Heritage Foundation had done . . . I worked with the people from Heritage at that time, and then I introduced it to some of the legislators here" (Interview September 2013). Republican support for a small business insurance exchange increased in 2008 when House Minority Leader Tom Taylor, House Minority Whip Keith Gardner, and staff member Matt Kennicott visited Utah to learn about the new exchange being developed in Utah (Interviews September 2013). Gardner and Kennicott would ultimately play major roles in the debate over an exchange as key advisors to Governor Susana Martinez. Their vision of an ideal exchange was developed during this period.

Democrats did not support the exchange bills of 2007 and 2008, not necessarily out of opposition to the concept of an exchange, but because they were hoping for a more comprehensive reform. Governor Bill Richardson was planning on running for president and wanted to pass a bill leading to universal coverage. His original proposal contained many of the elements that would later be included in the ACA, such as an individual mandate, an employer mandate, and low-cost government-subsidized insurance plans (NM Health Care Reform Leadership Team 2010). Compared to Governor Richardson's proposal, Democrats and consumer advocates saw the small business exchange as a way for Republicans to weaken more significant proposals. They considered Republican proposals for an exchange as simply a way to sell insurance, doing very little to expand coverage (Interviews 2013–2014). One Democratic Senator described it as "a glorified brokerage for insurance companies" (Interview September 2014).

The partisan politics surrounding an exchange shifted with the passage of the ACA. As one conservative leader described, "Some Republicans at that point were hesitant because they saw it as a mandate from Obama. Those of us who had been working on it awhile knew it wasn't; that this was actually a pretty decent idea" (Interview September 2013). At the same time, Democrats who had been reluctant to support an exchange were now fully supportive (Interviews 2013–2014).

So why did it take three years for the state to decide to create an exchange? One of the most important moments took place before the debate even really began, with the election of Governor Susanna Martinez in 2010 and the Democrat's majority in the House shrinking to four seats. Yet even with a Republican governor, the debate in New Mexico was never really about whether to do an exchange, but what type of exchange to establish.

The lack of a strong Tea Party presence in New Mexico gave consumer groups greater latitude to push for what they saw as a more favorable model of an exchange. But procedural rules gave the governor and supporters of a market-oriented exchange a major advantage. Even though states had between the ACA's passage in March 2010 until the beginning of an exchange's open enrollment in October 2013, the New Mexico legislature only had two 60-day windows to decide which path to take.

Democrats ultimately won the legislative fight, though ironically, the exchange that was actually implemented closely resembles Governor Martinez's preferences. This chapter traces the evolution of the debate in New Mexico, following the same chronological outline as the other case study chapters (see Appendix D for a timeline of key events in New Mexico).

MARCH 2010—DECEMBER 2010

Governor Bill Richardson (D) responded enthusiastically throughout 2010 to the ACA's passage. As he prepared to leave office, he laid the foundation for whoever succeeded him in 2011 to follow through with its implementation. Grants were sought and work groups convened, with particular attention paid to the creation of a state-based health insurance exchange.

Exchange Planning under Richardson

The task force convened by Governor Richardson issued a report on July 1, 2010, recommending that New Mexico establish its own exchange rather than using a federally operated exchange and that it should be a highly regulated active purchaser instead of the more open clearinghouse model. The report stated, "While some states have developed exchanges that merely serve as a market organization and distribution center for health care plans, it is recommended that New Mexico develop a strong exchange that promotes competition between plans based on quality and price in a way that is transparent to consumers" (NM Health Care Reform Leadership Team 2010). A legislative task force made similar recommendations later in the year (Armstrong 2010).

In July, Governor Richardson created the New Mexico Office of Health Care Reform within the Human Services Department (NM Executive Order 2010-032). This office took the lead on planning activities, including receiving a $1 million grant from the federal government to conduct stakeholder engagement. By the end of the year, the Office of Health Care Reform had commissioned thirteen studies and spent $600,000 of this planning grant (Coughlin 2012).

Many participants describe these work groups as valuable for bringing stakeholders together and making positions known. Businesses, insurers, and consumer advocates all participated. Although there was disagreement over whether the exchange should be an active purchaser or clearinghouse, it became clear that there was consensus in favor of maintaining state control (Interviews 2013–2014). Even so, not everyone agreed that these meetings were worthwhile. As one insurance broker described:

> Richardson was a classic decision-maker by consensus. He didn't like decisions being made in vacuums. So he would create work groups and committees. It was absolutely exhausting and absolutely worthless. More work was done and put up on a shelf and never done anything with it than anything I've seen in my entire career. . . . Nothing ever came out of any of them. (Interview September 2013)

These meetings and reports occurred against the backdrop of uncertainty over who would replace Bill Richardson as governor. Had Democratic Lieutenant Governor Diane Denish won, as many expected, the work group recommendations likely would have served as the foundation for the ACA's implementation. Instead, Republican Susanna Martinez won with 53% of the vote. Health reform was not a major issue in the 2010 gubernatorial race. Governor-Elect Martinez made generic statements opposing the ACA, but gave no indication of how she would approach an exchange (Interviews 2013–2014).

On December 27, 2010, Richardson's Office of Health Care Reform prepared a transition plan for the incoming Martinez administration. One recommendation was to pass legislation in the 2011 session to create a quasi-governmental exchange with active purchaser powers, and with a board excluding anyone having a conflict of interest, including insurers, agents, and brokers. The plan recommended moving the Office of Health Care Reform to the governor's office and hiring a director who reports directly to the governor (New Mexico Office of Health Reform). As governor, Susana Martinez did neither.

JANUARY 2011—NOVEMBER 2011

The second implementation period was dominated by two events: the 2011 legislative session, in which Governor Martinez vetoed legislation that would have created an active purchaser exchange, and the interim period before the next legislative session in which her office took steps to create a different type of exchange.

2011 Legislative Session

Multiple exchange bills were introduced early in the 2011 session, all by Democrats and all with minimal input from the new governor. Representative Danice Picraux and Senator Dede Feldman introduced in each chamber parallel legislation that would have created an active purchaser exchange with a consumer-oriented board (New Mexico House Bill [HB] 33, 2011; New Mexico Senate Bill [SB] 38, 2011). Senator George Muñoz introduced a less prescriptive bill that provided a framework, but let the exchange's board decide how it would operate (New Mexico Senate Bill [SB] 370, 2011).

Two of the chief negotiators during the session were not legislators or industry leaders. Gail Evans of the New Mexico Center on Law and Poverty represented consumer advocates pushing for an active purchaser exchange, and J. R. Damron was a prominent Republican pushing for a clearinghouse exchange. Legislators have limited staff compared to the governor and meet too infrequently to develop expertise on the nuances of issues. As a result, they found it advantageous to let trusted allies sort out the policy details.

Evans initially supported Representative Picraux's bill, though it never made it out of the House. Muñoz's bill suffered the same fate in the Senate, making it through committee but never receiving a vote on the floor. The focus shifted to Senator Feldman's bill, which one disappointed Democrat described as initially "a very progressive bill" that was "much less than that" when it ultimately passed the Senate (Interview September 2013). The bill did not receive a vote on the Senate Floor until March 2, which is very late in the session for a bill to have a realistic chance of passage in a second chamber (New Mexico Senate Roll Call #215 2011).

The process in the House was even more contentious, with Republicans refusing to compromise. House Democrats needed every member to fall in line since the recent election had dramatically shrunk the size of their majority. The bill SB 38 passed the House Consumer and Public Affairs Committee by a party-line 3 to 2 vote on March 10. A week later, it passed the House Appropriations and Finance Committee on a 10 to 8 vote also split along party lines (NM SB 38 2011). Supporters of the original bill say that the only good thing left after making its way through two chambers was a conflict of interest provision preventing insurers, brokers, and doctors from serving on the board of directors. The only reason this survived was because most people expected the Obama administration to include such a provision in its forthcoming regulations anyway (Interviews September 2013).[2] There were also concerns over how much an exchange would cost, but US Senator Jeff Bingaman (D-NM) wrote each state legislator a letter attempting to reassure them that the federal government would follow through with its promised share (Williams 2011).

By the time SB 38 made it to the House floor, leadership had commitments from enough conservative Democrats to ensure passage if the vote could be called at the right moment (Interviews September 2014). When it is in session, the New Mexico legislature technically meets 24 hours per day, each day of the week. By contrast, the legislatures in Idaho, Michigan, and Mississippi conduct business for a few hours per day when in session, adjourning until a set time the next business day. As a result, supportive interest groups played a role beyond the conventional lobbying work of convincing legislators, providing data to allies, and taking head counts—they helped the House leadership keep track of who was physically in the chamber at any given time (Interviews September 2013).

Democrats sensed their opportunity late in the evening of Friday March 18, knowing they had thirty-four votes in favor and noticing that three Republicans were absent because they were sick or otherwise unable to make it to the floor. A roll call was announced shortly after midnight on the morning of March 19, the second to last day of the 2011 legislative session. Thus, SB 38 passed by three votes (NM 2011 Roll Call #3293). As one supporter described, "It was amazing how [Speaker Ben Luján] managed to finagle it to call it up at the precise moment when there were just enough votes in the room to pass it" (Interview September 2013).

It was not clear how Governor Martinez would react. A few weeks earlier, she said she was not sure she would be willing to sign any of the exchange bills introduced that session (Jennings 2011). After the bill passed, she took three weeks before finally deciding to veto it. She argued in her veto message that the bill was premature and, "legislators ignored my administration's attempts to address the concerns I had with this particular piece of legislation" (Martinez 2011). The only concern she specified in this message was the cost of maintaining a self-sustaining exchange, though legislators say the biggest complaint they heard from her was over the composition of the board (Interviews 2013–2014). Senator Feldman, the original sponsor of the bill that passed, explained, "It wasn't just a question of who gets to be on the board, but who gets to appoint the board. The governor wanted more power. We weren't really that far apart. It was unfortunate that she vetoed it" (Interview September 2013).

A number of people interviewed attribute Governor Martinez's decision to the people around her. Sometimes this explanation is given as a matter of fact disagreement over policy between people on different sides of the political spectrum. Her new chief of staff, Keith Gardner, was a strong supporter of creating an exchange modeled after Utah and testified against other types of exchange bills. He therefore encouraged Governor Martinez to veto any bill not resembling Utah's.

Others are more cynical in their assessment of who was advising her. A Democratic legislator believes "the insurance industry got to her" (Interview September 2013). One person who did not support the bill said that Governor Martinez was completely disorganized in the early months of her administration and did not understand what was in front of her (Interview September 2013). A supporter of the bill echoed this comment and added that the people she listened to most were more focused on politics than on policy (September 2013). Another legislator shared this view, explaining, "Keith Gardner was not a friend to the advocacy groups supporting an exchange. It was very clear to me that it was going to get vetoed" (Interview September 2013) simply because it had the support of consumer groups. Another person added, "Keith Gardner understands enough to be dangerous" (Interview October 2013).

Multiple people attribute the decision to political operative Jay McCleskey, the person credited with "discovering" Susana Martinez and convincing her to run for governor. Emblematic of his power within the Martinez administration as the person running her political action committee SusanaPAC, McCleskey is nicknamed "the 5th floor," a play on the fact that New Mexico's governor is regularly referred to as "the 4th floor," given the office's location on the top level of the Capitol Building (Interviews 2013). In other words, his power exceeds the governor's. He was not publicly involved in the debate over an exchange, but was said to be an important advocate of the veto behind the scenes (Interviews 2013–2014).

Democrats in the legislature say there was no real discussion of attempting to override her veto. One Representative explained, "We are wimps and the math isn't there" (Interview September 2013). As SB 38 had barely passed the House, it was very unlikely that enough votes could be secured to override the veto. There was little the legislature could do over the following nine months to work on implementing the ACA besides holding information-gathering interim committee meetings. If any progress was going to be made, it was up to Governor Martinez and her administration.

Interim Session

Martinez was among the twenty-nine Republican governors who signed a letter in July 2011 calling for the full repeal of the ACA (Olson 2011). Some of the media coverage surrounding Governor Martinez's veto portrayed her as an ideologue opposed to Obamacare. She was described in the same category as Bobby Jindal of Louisiana, Rick Scott of Florida, and Sam Brownback of Kansas, who had returned federal grant dollars in protest and vowed not to implement the ACA.

Yet, interviews with key players reveal a different picture. Governor Martinez was taking, or at least allowing people in her administration to take, important steps toward creating an exchange. Unlike in Mississippi, Michigan, and Idaho, there were no loud Republican voices within New Mexico calling for Governor Martinez to oppose an exchange, despite Republican legislative gains in the 2010 elections. One advisor to Governor Martinez describes the summer of 2011 by saying that even though she had just vetoed the exchange bill, "The Office of Health Reform was still working on stakeholder meetings and planning activities. They were holding interagency meetings. The work was very much moving forward on a state-based exchange, regardless of what the narrative was outside the administration" (Interview September 2013).

One of the most important steps taken that summer was the appointment of Dan Derksen to lead the Office of Health Reform. Dr. Derksen was a Republican leading the New Mexico Medical Society and had recently been a Robert Wood Johnson Foundation (RWJF) Congressional Fellow in the office of US Senator Jeff Bingaman in DC (Robert Wood Johnson Foundation 2011, Jennings 2012). Appointed in August, Derksen moved quickly to put together an application for a level 1 establishment grant before the September 30 deadline. The application requested $34 million, with most of the money going to IT development. Governor Martinez wrote a letter of support to Secretary Kathleen Sebelius, saying, "I am pleased to endorse" the grant application (New Mexico Dept of Human Services). Derksen also made it known that he planned on applying for a much larger level 2 establishment grant by the March 2012 deadline (Interviews 2013–2014).

The reaction from supporters of an exchange was mixed. They interpreted the grant application as evidence that planning was moving forward again. One legislator describes, "When, Dr. Derksen set to work immediately and got one of the early grants, we were off and running. It looked very promising" (Interview February 2014). A consumer advocate said they had expected nothing to happen, but, "When the agency got the grants, we thought 'oh, maybe they are going to do an exchange. She vetoed the bill, but now they are getting money and doing shit'" (Interview September 2013).

At the same time, advocates did not like that the application was written under the premise that the state's exchange would be established within the Health Insurance Alliance. The Alliance was a nonprofit created in 1994 as the conservative answer to "New Mexicare," a proposal in 1993 that would have created a single-payer healthcare system. The legislature rejected New Mexicare and instead created the Alliance in the face of aggressive lobbying from small businesses and the insurance industry (Ortiz y Pino 1993, Quick 1994). The board was dominated by insurance companies, causing Carol Miller, a New Mexican public health expert who had served on President Clinton's health reform task force, to describe the Alliance as "a total waste of time. The whole point of health care reform is that we have to get the insurance companies out of health care, not make it more convenient for them to be in it. . . . The five insurers represented on the board will write the plans and help set the rates. The small business alliance is an insurer's pipe dream" (Peterson 1994).

Insurance companies were not enthusiastic about the bills in 2007 and 2008 (New Mexico House Bill [HB] 1045, 2007; New Mexico Senate Bill [SB] 976, 2007) to build an exchange through the Alliance. As the head of government affairs for one of the major insurers describes, "There were a lot of good points to that bill and we generally supported what [Damron] was trying to do. But we thought that the way it was structured was duplicative of the Alliance, but also just in general of what insurance carriers are supposed to do anyway. Anytime there are duplicative efforts, there are duplicative costs. That was our take back then" (Interview September 2013). Their position shifted with the passage of the ACA in 2010. They did not suddenly love the idea of an exchange, but if one was going to be created, the Alliance was seen as a good model because it ensured they would play a leading role in its operation (Interviews 2013–2014).

Opponents of running an insurance exchange through the Alliance were worried for this exact reason. They feared that it would be controlled by insurers and the governor, rather than being favorable to consumers (Coughlin 2012). The fight during the 2011 session had been over this very issue, and many felt frustrated that the governor was circumventing the legislature (Interviews 2013–2014). Yet there was little they could do at this point to oppose Governor Martinez.

All indications were that she would soon sign an executive order to formally create the exchange as part of the Alliance (Interviews 2013–2014). The announcement in November 2011 that the US Supreme Court would hear the case against the ACA changed the dynamic in ways that were at first subtle, but that would ultimately deepen the divide between the Republicans in the executive branch and the Democrats in the legislative branch.

NOVEMBER 2011—JUNE 2012

The legislature met for thirty days from January 17–February 16, 2012, but the session was of no consequence in the debate over an exchange. Procedural rules stipulate that the legislature is only allowed to consider two kinds of legislations in even numbered years: (1) bills reacting to a special message from the governor, and (2) bills directly connected to the budget. The governor sent no such message on the exchange, and there was no precedent for passing this type of legislation in a budget session. One Democratic legislator explained, "We've tried that in the past, but it hasn't worked" (Interview September 2013). Some were frustrated that Governor Martinez had not made it possible to pass exchange legislation, but were not surprised given her administration's position that it could create an exchange through the Alliance by executive order.

With the legislature out of the picture, the most important actions in late 2011 and early 2012 took place behind the scenes. Request for proposals (RFPs) were sent out by the Office of Health Reform so vendors could bid on different aspects of building the exchange IT. Firms were chosen and contracts were written, waiting for the signature of Human Services Department Secretary Sidonie Squier (Interviews 2013–2014). Dan Derksen was nearly ready to submit the state's application for a level 2 establishment grant of more than $100 million to pay for the first year of the exchange's operation. The Centers for Medicare and Medicaid Services (CMS) was consulted and indicated support for the grant as long as a legal framework was developed to create the exchange—that is, legislation or an executive order. Governor Martinez's office went over multiple drafts of an executive order that it said was to soon be issued (Interviews 2013–2014). The RFPs released in March 2012 indicated that the state planned on applying for a level 2 grant by July, implying the executive order would be signed by then.

Instead, Derksen resigned suddenly in late March, the grant application was never submitted, and progress stalled. Different people have different explanations for Derksen's departure. People within the Martinez administration say they wanted more time to review the grant before it was submitted and that this frustrated Derksen. The governor's office released a statement praising him for moving "this administration forward in setting up a framework to establish a statewide health insurance exchange in the face of great uncertainty from the federal government" (Jennings 2012).

People outside the administration saw Derksen's departure as a worrisome sign. As one advocate said, "Dan was a very serious thinker about health care reform. The Office of Health Care Reform was in good hands. The fact that he left so suddenly, and it was sudden—we had a phone call scheduled for next week—that always raises questions" (Jennings 2012). A Democratic legislator said, "It was almost like the guillotine dropped in March of 2012 when [Derksen] was dumped. The Governor's office announced that he left his position, but it was pretty clear that he was dumped" (Interview February 2014).

Many identify Human Services Secretary Sidonie Squier and Martinez advisor Jay McCleskey as the people behind Derksen's departure. One person closely involved described their view of what happened behind the scenes. When the executive order and the $100-million grant application were ready to go, "I think the light went off in Squier's head that this was really going to happen. She was doing everything she could to block it, but it was moving forward" (Interview March 2014). The same week that the Supreme Court heard oral arguments on the ACA's case, Squier told Derksen to halt activity on the exchange. Derksen immediately resigned, saying that Squier and McCleskey were blocking progress and that he did not want to be held responsible when the exchange did not work (Interviews 2013–2014).

Derksen's resignation from the Office of Health Care Reform would not be the final chapter in the debate over an insurance exchange, but it was an important turning point. Planning activities within the Martinez administration completely stopped. The governor did not sign the executive order creating an exchange. The level 2 establishment grant application was never submitted. Martinez did nothing with the $34-million level 1 grant that had already been received. Contracts with chosen vendors were not signed, and no action was taken on the responses to new RFPs that had been issued. It appeared that the state would take no action on the exchange until after the Supreme Court ruling (Interviews 2013–2014).

There is no evidence that this shift was driven by interest groups. Many of the state's industry leaders opposed the ACA and hoped the Court would overturn the law, but they preferred state control of the exchange and wanted the state to be ready in case the law survived its challenges (Interviews 2013–2014). Instead, it seemed that New Mexico was being swept up in national conservative politics. Martinez's advisers did not want to be associated with any aspect of Obamacare during this crucial period in which the law was being considered by the Supreme Court and a major part of the 2012 elections.

JULY 2012—OCTOBER 2013

In July 2012 the venue for the debate over an exchange shifted to the legislature's Interim Health and Human Services Committee. Interim committees have no formal powers, but are where much of the legislating takes place. The hope is that consensus on which issues to prioritize and which bills to support can be developed even before a session begins. The Interim Health and Human Services Committee met monthly from July to December 2012, with an insurance exchange being on the agenda more often than any other issue (NM Legislative Health and Human Services Interim Committee 2012).

Human Services Department Secretary Sidonie Squier testified at the July 9 meeting held in the city of Truth or Consequence just two weeks after the Supreme Court's ruling was released. She indicated that the administration was still planning on moving forward with creating an exchange through the Alliance and had hired Leavitt Partners to take the lead on planning efforts. When asked why the Department was not spending any of the $34 million level 1 grant, particularly after RFPs had been sent out and contracts prepared, Squier responded that the contracts written by Dan Derksen were being rewritten by Leavitt Partners because "the original request for proposals did not meet New Mexico's needs." The committee pushed back on this point, quoting her intention to create an exchange "designed by New Mexico." One member observed that Dr. Derksen was from New Mexico, had worked in New Mexico, and had worked in Congress for a New Mexican Senator, but that the Department was rejecting his work and hiring a Utah consultant instead to set up the exchange. Squier replied, "Dr. Derksen had no experience working on an exchange and Leavitt does" (NM Legislative Health and Human Services Interim Committee 2012).

Another point of debate at the July meeting was whether an exchange could be established without legislation. The committee complained that the Martinez administration was excluding the legislature from its planning. Secretary Squier promised to communicate with legislators and conceded that legislation would probably be needed at some point to amend the statute governing the Alliance, even if the legal authority for the exchange was established by executive order (NM Legislative Health and Human Services Interim Committee 2012).

An exchange came up again at the September 11 meeting held in Las Vegas, New Mexico. Democrat Senator Dede Feldman asked the attorney general's office to address whether Governor Martinez had the authority to create an exchange by executive order. Assistant Attorney General

Mark Reynolds explained his office's opinion, "such action is likely to be unconstitutional" because it would violate the separation of powers provision of the New Mexico Constitution (NM Legislative Health and Human Services Interim Committee 2012). Reynolds's letter to the committee cited an incident from 1998 in which Governor Gary Johnson vetoed legislation to implement Clinton's welfare reform, and then used an executive order to implement the reform a different way. The legislature sued and the state Supreme Court found the governor's attempt at unilateral action to be unconstitutional. Reynolds concluded that the facts in this case "are analogous to the situation we would have should the Governor create a health insurance exchange by executive order" (Reynolds 2012).

Democrats reacted confidently to this opinion from the attorney general's office that Martinez could not create an exchange without legislation. "We had already passed a bill that she had vetoed, so we already had her," said a House Democrat (Interview September 2013). With the help of the Center on Law and Poverty, Democrats hired a private law firm to prepare a lawsuit. One of the legislators involved in preparing the suit explained, "When we did that, Matt Kennicott and others [from the Martinez administration] reached out and said 'let's work together.' So they stopped what they were doing with the Alliance. . . . The lawsuit never got filed; but it was ready at the drop of a hat" (Interview September 2013). Another legislator involved noted the potential for this plan to backfire, observing, "We did have a little bit of a gun pointed to her head, but we had an even bigger gun to our head. If we had sued it would have been delayed, and we wouldn't have had a state-based exchange anyway" (Interview February 2014). An advisor to Governor Martinez described this period in more diplomatic terms, saying "The governor said she didn't think we needed to have legislation, but in good faith I'm willing to talk and see what good ideas we can come up with. Maybe we'll come up with something better" (Interview September 2013).

Two members of the Martinez administration spoke at the final interim committee meeting on November 27 in Santa Fe: Secretary Squier and Milton Sanchez, the new Director of the Office of Health Care Reform. They explained that the Obama administration had extended a key exchange deadline to December 14 and that New Mexico would submit a declaration letter and blueprint plan by that date. The committee voted to endorse an exchange bill, even though it would do so through the Alliance.

Senator Dede Feldman supported this new bill, saying, "I thought that was good because I wanted a road to compromise" (Interview September 2013). As the chair of the interim committee and the author of the exchange bill vetoed by Governor Martinez in 2011, her support carried a lot of weight. Foreshadowing the tensions that would erupt in the coming legislative session, not everyone agreed with her. A consumer advocate who wanted a strong exchange explained that this bill was awful, and, "now it was going to be hard for us to do anything because the Democratic leadership had endorsed a crappy exchange bill before the session even started" (Interview September 2013).

The fact that Senator Feldman and Representative Picraux were retiring before the start of the session just weeks away injected further uncertainty into the debate. Democrats talked during the last interim committee meeting about who would carry the mantle in their place. They explained that almost by default it fell to Jerry Ortiz y Pino in the Senate and Mimi Stewart in the House. This group appointed Gail Evans of the Center on Law and Poverty as their lead negotiator on an exchange. In the weeks leading up to the start of the 2013 legislative session, Evans met regularly with Matt Kennicott of the Human Services Department and Milton Sanchez of the Office of Health Care Reform (Interviews 2013–2014).

2013 Legislative Session

The US Supreme Court's surprise decision to make the Medicaid expansion optional put another controversial Obamacare issue onto the agenda for the 2013 legislative session. In mid-January, Governor Martinez announced support for expansion. This showed she could step away from intense partisan national politics under the right circumstances. She explained in her State of the State speech on January 21, 2014, "I wasn't a supporter of ObamaCare. But under its mandate we had a choice whether to expand Medicaid using federal funds. We chose to expand Medicaid because it was the right thing to do for New Mexico" (Martinez 2014a).

Expansion was also good politics in New Mexico. A poll three months earlier found that 52% of New Mexicans supported expansion, compared to 33% who were opposed (Associated Press [AP] 2012). As an incumbent governor, she was less likely to receive a serious primary challenge for the 2014 election. Now having expanded Medicaid, she had taken away a major attack Democratic challengers were likely to make.

Expanding Medicaid increased her leverage in the exchange debate while also lowering its stakes. Fewer people would be affected by the exchange than by Medicaid, and Democrats would have a hard time portraying her as an ideologue on the exchange when she had just expanded Medicaid. Even so, both sides continued to aggressively push for their model of an exchange to be adopted.

Four exchange bills were introduced in the early days of the 2013 legislative session, two in the House and two in the Senate. Democrats were weakened by not better coordinating and compromising before the start of the session. Once again, the main differences between the bills were whether the exchange would be an active purchaser or a clearinghouse, who could sit on the board of directors, and how many seats on the board would be appointed by the governor and the legislature. Negotiations between Gail Evans and the Martinez administration continued, with Democratic legislators and consumer advocates optimistic it would lead to compromise. By late January they believed that a deal had been reached and that the governor would support a compromise bill. One advocate explained that Gail Evans and Mimi Stewart "spent hours working with the fourth floor [i.e., the governor's office], just working on that bill. It got watered down, but they felt it was acceptable."

However, if there had in fact been an agreement with the governor's staff, it would soon be off. Another consumer advocate describes, "Matt [Kennicott] comes to a meeting and at the very end, when we thought we were done, he has changes to the bill that he now wanted that completely changed the entire agreement. . . . The language that he wanted was language that Keith Gardner was insisting on. It was very strong no active purchaser language" (Interview September 2013). A House Democrat involved in the negotiations adds, "after working with us for three weeks, they killed the bill" (Interview September 2013).

Representative Stewart went forward anyway with a bill reflecting what she understood the agreement to be with the Martinez administration. One consumer advocate described this as a smart move. "It wasn't the perfect bill, but it was the bill we thought we could live with, including Matt Kennicott and all those folks we were negotiating with. It was everything we had all agreed to" (Interview September 2013). House bill 168 narrowly made it through the House Health, Government, and Indian Affairs committee on a 6–5 vote (NM House Health, Government & Indian Affairs Committee 2013a) and then the House Judiciary Committee on a vote of 9–6 (NM House Judiciary Committee 2013).

The bill then faced an uphill battle on the House floor, though not necessarily because of politics related to health reform. A number of legislators held a grudge against Representative Stewart for a role she had played the previous year in a fight over the education budget and refused to vote for any of her bills. They approached other Democrats who supported HB 168 and explained, "it's not your message, it's your messenger" (Interview September 2013). The bill was defeated 30–39 (NM House Roll Call #3928). It may not have mattered anyway, as the governor's office was telling supporters of an exchange that Governor Martinez would veto this bill. If they wanted New Mexico to retain control of its insurance exchange, they needed to defeat Stewart's bill and find an alternative (Interviews 2013–2014).

In the meantime, two bills were making their way through the Senate. The governor indicated she would support a bill written by Senator Benny Shendo. An advisor to Governor Martinez explained, "his bill wasn't perfect, but a major selling point was that it wasn't an active purchaser" (Interview September 2013). Some were skeptical of Senator Shendo, because he was only a few weeks into his first term in the legislature and had no prior experience in health policy. Still, his bill seemed to be the best path toward compromise with the governor.

A key turning point occurred in early March, when Senator Jerry Ortiz y Pino merged his bill with Senator Shendo's, dropping expectations of an active purchaser exchange in the process. Senator Ortiz y Pino was viewed by many in the legislature as a progressive champion and as the standard bearer on this issue since Dede Feldman's retirement. His support for Senator Shendo's bill split those pushing for a state-based exchange. The Center on Law and Poverty, Representative Stewart, and a handful of others still wanted an active purchaser exchange. One supporter of this approach explained, "Jerry's role really doomed us. When he got behind a bad bill, I couldn't get anybody's attention because if Jerry think it's OK—he's like the most progressive guy in the building, you must just be real extreme" (Interview September 2013). Senate leadership decided, "if Jerry's OK with this, then we're OK with this" (Interview September 2013). The Center on Law and Poverty went so far as to advocate against Senator Shendo's bill, saying that New Mexico would be better off with a federally run exchange.

The merger between Senator Shendo and Senator Ortiz y Pino occurred with only ten days left in the session, putting great pressure on the final negotiations. One person involved explained, "It became clear that the governor didn't have sticking points if the insurers would agree, so we knew we had to get the insurers . . .. They had differences of opinion among them, so these were tedious meetings. The lobbyists kept having to run out and call their handlers" (Interview February 2014).

Insurers were united in their desire for opposing active purchaser language and for increasing their representation on the board. At the same time, they worried about a scenario in which there were not enough seats for each of the major players. As one insurance leader described, "The thought was that we definitely want representation, but if it's just one seat, it could be a bad thing because what if it is [our competitor]?" (Interview

September 2013). Ultimately a compromise was reached with two seats going to the industry, with half of the board being appointed by the governor and half selected by the legislature. This was not as many seats as insurers wanted, but they decided it was better than having an active purchaser exchange or giving up control to the federal government. The insurance industry united behind SB 221 (Interviews September 2013).

The bill was then rushed through the Senate, passing the Corporations and Transportation Committee 8–2 on Friday March 8, amended on the Senate floor Sunday March 10, and passed 36–5 on Monday March 11 (New Mexico Senate Corporations and Transportation Committee 2013, New Mexico Senate Bill [SB] 221).

House Democrats were divided over how to respond at this point. There were only five days left in the session, leading some to conclude, "We have to get something. It's late in the session, so you have to get something on her desk or she's going to do this by executive order or blame the Democrats" for a federal exchange (Interview September 2013). Even so, with House Republicans united behind Senator Shendo's bill, it was clear it could pass if leadership could navigate the bill through the process on time. The bill was sent to a committee chaired by someone from the same city as Senator Shendo, where it passed 11–0 on Thursday March 14 (NM House Health, Government & Indian Affairs Committee 2013b). The bill was then approved by the full House by a vote of 61–7 on Friday March 15, the next to last day of the session (New Mexico Senate Roll Call #4237 2011). The only "no" votes came from Democrats, who supported the concept of an exchange but did not think this bill went far enough.

There was no serious talk within Governor Martinez's office of vetoing SB 221. An advisor to Governor Martinez confirmed this point, comparing the legislative process in 2013 to the debate in 2011 when the key bill needed to be voted on after midnight to ensure passage. Referring to 2013, this advisor said, "Towards the end, surprisingly, I didn't notice any political games being played. By the time we were done with this, everyone had given up so much, and everyone knew that everyone had given up so much, there were really no games. It was sort of, we need to get this done" (Interview September 2013). And with that, New Mexico had decided to create its own health insurance exchange.

The most striking difference in this debate compared to what happened in Idaho, Michigan, and Mississippi was the lack of Tea Party mobilization. Skocpol and Williamson (2012) list New Mexico as one of the fifteen states in the nation with more than 4–6 Tea Party organizations per million people. However, the Tea Party played almost no role in the debate over whether or not to create an exchange in New Mexico. They did not show up to legislative meetings at anywhere near the levels seen in other states in my sample, nor were they active online. Nobody interviewed cited the Tea Party as a major force in the debate, with most people emphasizing that the Tea Party is not very strong in New Mexico politics (Interviews 2013–2014). The Tea Party is seen as having some strength in the southern part of the state, such as having multiple seats on the Rio Rancho City Council. However, the population in this part of the state is extremely sparse, making it difficult for groups to organize. Most of these people live too far from the capital in Santa Fe to consistently influence the legislative process.

Further evidence of the Tea Party's weakness, or perhaps a contributing factor, is the lack of a strong conservative think tank organization. There is the Rio Grande Foundation led by Paul Gessing, but it does not have nearly the same level of influence in state politics as the Idaho Freedom Foundation, Michigan's Mackinac Center for Public Policy, and the Mississippi Center for Public Policy. The Rio Grande Foundation did not take an active role in arguing against an exchange. For example, the Rio Grande Foundation did not publish a single report or blog post during the 2013 legislative relevant to the exchange debate. This left a leadership and an information void weakening any attempt at Tea Party mobilization against an exchange.

Post-Session

As the dust settled on a contentious three-year debate over whether New Mexico would run an insurance exchange and who would be put in charge, policymakers went to work to meet tight deadlines ahead of the beginning of open enrollment on October 1. J. R. Damron, the 2006 Republican nominee for governor and the man largely credited with being the first to push for an exchange in New Mexico, was named Chair of the Board of Directors. Governor Martinez used her five appointments to select leaders from the insurance industry, small businesses, hospitals, and providers. Republican leadership in the House and Senate had one appointment each, which they used to select hospital leaders.

Supporters of a strong exchange feel that Democratic leadership in each chamber squandered their appointments, selecting people too closely aligned with insurers and hospitals (Interviews 2013–2014). One Democrat who supported the final compromise legislation said, "The irony was that one of the things we didn't back down on was that the legislative leaders needed to appoint people—but they basically just appointed twins to who the governor appointed. . . . We blew our appointments on hospitals" (Interview February 2014). Another referenced Representative Mimi's Stewart's frustration with SB 221, saying "Mimi was very angry, saying it would have been better to have no bill at all. Now, looking at the composition of our exchange, I think she might have been right" (Interview September 2013).

The disappointment was compounded by the fact that one of the first decisions the board made was to give up control to the federal government. Jon Kingsdale spoke at the first board meeting on April 29 about the challenges the board would face in building an exchange on time. Kingsdale is a Boston-based consultant who was one of the architects of the Massachusetts exchange in 2006 and was working with many other states in establishing an exchange. He explained that the state would likely be ready to run the exchange by 2015, but it was too late to be ready for 2014's open enrollment just five months away (Warwick 2013).

Instead of trying to build both the individual and small-business exchange in such a short period of time, the Board decided to focus on the SHOP exchange and rely on the federal exchange for the individual market. One board member explained that the state already had significant experience with the small business market from nearly twenty years of running the Alliance, and so it made sense to focus energies there (Interview September 2013).

Supporters of a robust New Mexico exchange describe it as frustratingly ironic that the outcome of years of debate so closely matches what they had opposed from the beginning. They pushed aggressively and won a legislative fight for state control, but still defaulted to the federal government. New Mexico's exchange would at least initially be focused on small businesses and based on the Alliance, exactly as Keith Gardner and others within the Martinez administration had originally wanted. Progressive Democrats fought hard for control over who would serve on the board but were disappointed when their leadership mostly used this power to appoint industry representatives. Stakeholders interviewed after October 1 also express deep frustration over the many problems surrounding the rollout of the federal website healthcare.gov. They lament that New Mexicans would not have been affected by the website's problems had state leaders acted sooner (Interviews 2013–2014). The irony is that years of fighting over who was empowered to decide and what type of exchange New Mexico would operate meant that the choice was made so late that the state had to give up control of its exchange anyway.

CHAPTER 6

Exchange Politics and the Future of Health Reform

Eminent retired political scientist Sidney Verba once remarked that if he were back in the classroom teaching on American government he would structure his course entirely around the ACA.[1] The law is a window into nearly every aspect of policymaking in the United States, including the internal workings of Congress, the relationship between the executive and legislative branches, the role of the courts, the challenges faced by executive branch agencies during implementation, federalism, and the differences between states. We can now add long-term stability and policy vulnerability as a result of subsequent elections to the list given Donald Trump's victory in 2016.

The opening sentence of this book described the ACA as the most significant health reform law enacted in generations. This is true. It is the largest increase of health insurance coverage in the United States since the creation of Medicare and Medicaid in 1965. The law has huge implications for a sector of the economy touching approximately 17% of the gross domestic product (Centers for Medicare and Medicaid Services 2016).

But it is also true that the ACA is a collection of disparate reforms (Béland, Rocco, and Waddan 2016) and that it is more like the culmination of decades of incremental reforms than a true overhaul of the US healthcare system. At the same time that they were celebrating the law's passage in March 2010, many Democrats were disappointed that this was the best they could get. They understood that the reform accepted and built on the current system rather than make fundamental changes. To them this was like putting Band-Aids on top of Band-Aids rather than truly solving the underlying problems. Even if fully successful, millions of people would still lack coverage and the government would not have significant leverage to keep spending down.

Congressional leaders appreciated that a health reform law would not accomplish anything if it was too liberal to win support from key stakeholders. The primary objective in designing the ACA was not necessarily to be the ideal solution to all the problems of US healthcare, but to thread the political needle to win enough support from Democrats to be passed while not attracting enough opposition from conservatives and key interest groups to be blocked.

Health insurance exchanges epitomize this mindset. This was a way to expand coverage that conservatives had supported for many years and in parts of the country as diverse as Massachusetts and Utah. As Ted Kennedy said at the bill-signing ceremony of the Massachusetts reform in 2006 that created the first statewide exchange, "when Kennedy and Romney support a piece of legislation, usually one of them hasn't read it" (Miga and LeBlance 2012). That they both could live with this approach made exchanges a major part of the political blueprint for national health reform. Democrats thought Republicans would appreciate that one of the centerpieces of the reform emphasized competition and market forces rather than something resembling a Canadian-style single-payer system. Senator Max Baucus, chair of the powerful Finance Committee, desperately hoped to win support from prominent Republicans such as Chuck Grassley and Orrin Hatch. He compromised away the public option, meaning the only plans sold on the exchange would be operated by private insurance companies rather than the government. To make the reform even more attractive to conservatives, Senate Democrats allowed for exchanges to be run at the state level rather than create a single national exchange run in Washington, DC. These compromises were enough to keep moderate Democrats on board, but they were not enough to win over even a single Republican in Congress.

Democrats were so focused on the politics of enactment that they paid less attention to anticipating the politics of implementation. One of the main reasons the launch of the exchanges was put off until 2014 was to keep the ten-year projections of the ACA's costs down because the Congressional Budget Office only estimates a bill's fiscal impact for a ten-year period. The fight over exchanges likely would have looked very different if states had only been given two years to launch an exchange instead of nearly four. State leaders would have complained about needing more time, but opponents would have had less opportunity to obstruct.

Supporters of the ACA figured they could worry about implementation later, and that these challenges would not matter anyway if they could not get the law through Congress in the first place. In any case, the politics of implementing exchanges were not expected to conflict with the politics that led to the ACA's passage. Any resistant states would be motivated by the preemption threat that the federal government would step in and run the exchange for them. State leaders want flexibility and would likely welcome the large amounts of money available from the federal government. Virtually every state was expected to create its own exchange.

This was a major miscalculation. Instead, opponents of the ACA used state flexibility to perpetuate obstructionism. State leaders initially cooperated on the exchanges while fighting the individual mandate and Medicaid expansion in court. But exchanges soon became the primary front in the larger battle to block the ACA. Leading opponents believed the federal government lacked the will and capacity to follow through with its threats. They could topple the mandate and the rest of the law if enough states refused to cooperate on the exchanges. Michael Cannon of the Cato Institute argued that refusing to pass legislation to set up an exchange is "the most powerful blow that a state can strike against Obamacare" (Kaplan 2012) and that officials who signed the lawsuit and accepted exchange grants were violating their oath of office by implementing a law they believed was unconstitutional (Mooney 2011).

The stories in Idaho, Michigan, Mississippi, and New Mexico illustrate what happened when opponents responded to this call to arms. Obscure procedural processes such as the Mississippi Personnel Services Contract Review Board's consideration of contracts with information technology (IT) vendors became part of a national fight against Obamacare. Opponents were amazingly effective, defeating the largest and most powerful interest groups in Michigan, Mississippi, and thirty-two other states.

WHAT HAPPENED?

The previous four chapters examined what happened in the last two states to opt for retaining control of an exchange (Idaho and New Mexico) and the two that came the closest but gave up control to the federal government (Michigan and Mississippi). Partisanship is a major element of the fight over exchanges in these states, but is not an adequate explanation for what happened. In other words, it is not enough to say that states led by Republicans decided not to create an exchange because they oppose Democrats and did not want to give President Obama any victories. This was certainly true for a lot of Republicans, but this simplistic view obscures the complexities of state politics and infighting on the right. The most significant division in many states was not between Democrats and Republicans, but within the Republican Party.

Four key factors explain what happened in these states: governors, the Tea Party, pockets of expertise, and leadership. How similar were these states to the rest of the country? I now turn to these four lessons to look at how they apply in these states and elsewhere. Most of the rest of the states were more like Michigan and Mississippi than like Idaho and New Mexico, but these latter states provide lessons on what could have been elsewhere.

Governors

First, governors were the most important actors within each state's fight over a health insurance exchange. Exchange legislation succeeded in Idaho largely because of the aggressive involvement of Governor Butch Otter. The other side of the same coin is that no state created an exchange without the backing of its governor, meaning an unsupportive governor could block an exchange. A state-run exchange was likely in Mississippi until Governor Phil Bryant got in the way. Elsewhere, the idea of creating an exchange in Florida and Louisiana was dead when governors Rick Scott and Bobby Jindal returned exchange grants. Some state leaders tried to keep an exchange alive against the governor's opposition, such as the independently elected Republican insurance commissioner Sandy Praeger in Kansas. Just as in Mississippi, there was very little she could do without the governor's support.

However, governors are not omnipotent. They vary significantly in their ability to advance an agenda (Berch 1992, Dukakis 2001, Beyle 2004). Rick Snyder's failure in Michigan shows that although necessary, a governor's support was not sufficient to create a state-based exchange. A handful of other governors, such as Democrat Bev Purdue in North Carolina and Democrat Pat Quinn of Illinois, supported a state-based exchange but were unable to win approval from their legislatures.

Governors are in a difficult position. They are largely held accountable by the public for state policies, yet legislators generally hold a monopoly on the power to introduce, amend, and pass laws. The only formal legislative power many governors hold is reactive—the ability to veto or sign bills passed by the legislature (Kousser and Phillips 2012). Even this authority varies by state, with forty-three having line item veto powers and thirty-seven being able to reduce the budget without legislative approval (Weissert and Weissert 2012).

Governors could have sidestepped the legislature entirely, creating an exchange by executive order. Governors in Kentucky, New York, and Rhode Island did just that after their legislatures failed to act. However, decisions made this way are vulnerable to being superseded by legislation or a change in gubernatorial power. The option of creating an exchange this way was technically available to every governor, though the political feasibility of this approach varied by state. At least eight state legislatures specifically forbade their governors from creating an exchange without its approval (Bagley and Jones 2015). As a result, governors supporting the creation of an exchange were severely limited in their formal powers to do so on their own.

Tea Party Power

Second, one of the most dramatic and unexpected aspects of the fight over health insurance exchanges is that traditionally powerful interest groups struggled so intensely against the Tea Party. Interviewees said they could not remember a single issue that united insurers, hospitals, providers, and consumer advocates like health insurance exchanges. This coalition included state-level groups typically aligned with Democrats and Republicans, which many hoped would give both sides cover. This book provides an in the trenches view of how the Tea Party operated within states to influence policy.

Interest groups were particularly active in support of an exchange in Idaho and Michigan. Groups in Michigan formed a loose coalition but did little to coordinate their efforts or to influence broader public opinion to the same degree as in Idaho. The same types of groups were involved in Mississippi but were not organized and engaging in coordinated lobbying to the same degree because the decisions were being made within the Department of Insurance rather than in the legislature. There was no need to lobby, since they were all at the table via the commissioner's advisory board.

Republican legislators were expected to be on the same page as the major interest groups in their states, since the exchange could be framed as a conservative idea, promoted competition, put people in private rather than public plans, and prevented federal preemption. The initial reaction from state-level Republicans suggested that this would work. They strongly opposed the individual mandate but saw the exchanges as a separate issue.

This changed profoundly after the 2010 elections in which the Tea Party played a major role in the rightward shift across the country.

Even so, many Republican governors in 2011 initially stood up to the Tea Party and still supported creating an exchange at the state level. Newly elected Governors Sam Brownback (R-KS), Mary Fallin (R-OK), and Scott Walker (R-WI) said they would accept the large innovator grants their states had received under the outgoing administrations. The Department of Health and Human Services (HHS) refused to award the $31.5 million grant to Kansas until Governor-Elect Brownback would commit to cooperate. The Obama administration wanted to spare itself the embarrassment of a new Republican governor refusing a grant and likely would have quietly denied the application if Brownback opposed. He gave his support in December 2010 before taking office, and the grant process continued (McClean 2010).

Governor Brownback—who had voted against the ACA a year earlier as a US Senator—told a frustrated Tea Party leader in Kansas that he accepted the grant "not to do Obamacare—I am not supportive of us doing Obamacare—but to use that to do an exchange that provides a market mechanism because I believe we can use more market forces in health care" (Cauthon 2011a). Governor Fallin told Oklahoman conservatives almost the same thing, that "[u]nlike the federal exchange Washington may try to force on us, the exchange we are trying to build offers a positive, free-market alternative to the big government, tax-and-spend plan that is the PPACA." Both returned their grants within months after Tea Party pressure intensified.

Scott Walker of Wisconsin held on a little longer. In December 2011 he announced that he was not returning the $38 million grant the state had received, but was stopping all planning. Meanwhile, Walker's opponents collected enough signatures to trigger a recall election. He was under enormous pressure to raise money from conservative leaders who adamantly opposed Obamacare (Pilkington 2016). Local Tea Party activists mailed him strings to symbolize the burden of receiving federal dollars. Governor Walker announced that he was giving back the innovator grant to HHS two days after the signatures were delivered (Jones, Bradley, and Oberlander 2014).

Governor Walker's reversal epitomizes an important aspect of the Tea Party's influence, that it is both grassroots and national (Skocpol and Williamson 2012). The Tea Party is a social movement that in many ways acts like an interest group. But it is different in that it is not a private interest with a hierarchal structure; there is no such thing as THE Tea Party. Instead, it is a collection of decentralized groups of activists. Their influence is largely through local politics, taking over county and precinct party organizations, regularly attending coffee hours and open houses held by local legislators. Walker seemed to be influenced both by the strings he received from grassroots activists and the need to ask wealthy conservatives around the state and around the nation for money.

Skocpol and Williamson (2012) explain that one of the most important consequences of the Tea Party movement has been the "populist boost given to professionally run and opulently funded right-wing advocacy organizations devoted to pushing ultra-free-market policies." Every state has a conservative think tank that also behaves much like an interest group, although they are not registered lobbyists in every case. These groups are loosely connected through a national umbrella organization, the State Policy Network.

External organizations played an important role in fueling the Tea Party's momentum and influence over the exchange debate. Conservative think tanks in Idaho (the Idaho Freedom Foundation), Michigan (the Mackinac Center for Public Policy), and Mississippi (the Mississippi Center for Public Policy) served as de facto leaders of the Tea Party. They did not lead meetings, but they educated citizen activists on the legislative process and provided the data and reports for them to use when contacting legislators or writing blog posts. National groups such as the Cato Institute, ALEC, the Heritage Foundation, and Americans for Prosperity played a similarly important role for these state groups and local activists, providing expertise—and in some cases money.

National conservative organizations did more to inspire and mobilize state-level groups than their liberal counterparts. Families USA focused more on the Medicaid expansion than on insurance exchanges. The most prominent state-level groups supporting an exchange were consumer advocates, who in most cases were part of the coalition of interest groups lobbying for local development of the exchange. But there was no liberal parallel to the Tea Party to do the grassroots work. Even if there had been, this issue may not have excited them much, since the consequence of inaction would have been a greater role for the Obama administration. This is a tradeoff that liberal advocates maybe could have lived with, particularly in states run by conservatives.

The Supreme Court's decision in *Citizens United v. Federal Elections Commission* (2010) made it easier for private donors to spend large amounts of money on campaigns. Billionaire brothers David and Charles Koch are two of the most prominent spenders in the political debate surrounding the ACA. They move money through multiple layers of organizations, making it very difficult to know exactly whom they are giving money to and how much they have spent (Barker and Meyer 2014). However, many states had conservative organizations with explicit or rumored connections to the Koch brothers. They are reportedly major contributors to the State Policy Network of conservative think tanks that became influential in many places (Kopan 2013), including Americans for Prosperity, which played a major role in opposing the exchange in Michigan.

The story of Sam Brownback in Kansas is another example of the informal but mutually reinforcing relationship between local Tea Party activists, state-level groups, and national conservative organizations. Governor Brownback appeared willing to resist pressure to return his grant until at least nineteen Kansan legislators, his chief of staff, and his policy director attended ALEC's annual meeting in early August. This was where a leader from the conservative Heritage Foundation called for "an unrelenting fight [against Obamacare]" with "house by house, floor by floor, room by room combat" (Mooney 2011). Governor Brownback announced he was refusing the grant money days after his staff members and legislators returned from the ALEC conference.

Pockets of Expertise

Third, differences in institutional design shape the decision-making process, which in turn greatly affects the political strategies and tactics used by stakeholders. Steinmo and Watts (1995) argue that scholars and pundits are missing the big picture in their analysis of why certain policies are adopted and others are not. Echoing the phrase used by Bill Clinton's strategists in 1992, they write, "it's the institutions, stupid." Similarly, Immergut (1992) writes that the analysis of policymaking should focus more explicitly on institutions and procedures, since "they select the groups whose views will be represented and they shape demands by changing the strategic environment in which the demands of groups are formulated."

Decision-making over the exchanges was particularly fragmented compared with other parts of the ACA, such as the Medicaid expansion, premium rate review, and the development of a medical loss ratio (Béland, Rocco, and Waddan 2016). This gave the Tea Party and opponents of an exchange a distinct advantage because it is much easier to block a proposal in fragmented policymaking than to successfully adopt one (Steinmo and Watts 1995, Oberlander 2003, Weissert and Weissert 2012). To succeed, proponents of an insurance exchange needed to win in multiple committees, multiple chambers, and multiple branches of government. On the other hand, Haislmaier's "house by house combat" only required succeeding at one of these veto points.

In some cases, policy legacies—similar to the concept of path dependence—changed the nature of the institutions themselves and affected the range of options available (Béland, Rocco, and Waddan 2016). The debate in New Mexico would have played out very differently if Governor Martinez and her allies did not believe they could use legislation passed in 1994 to create the type of exchange they wanted without approval from the legislature. The case in Mississippi was similar in that the debate was dramatically shaped by two unique aspects of the state's institutions: the insurance commissioner is independently elected and did not believe he needed the governor's support and a series of laws broadening the scope of the state's high risk pool may have allowed Commissioner Chaney to create an exchange without new legislation.

Certain institutional conditions enabled so-called "pockets of expertise" to play an important role in navigating this process (Burns et al. 2008). These are leaders with particular policy knowledge and political clout who were looked to for guidance. The Idaho case suggests that such pockets of expertise are a key part of a strategy to overcome Tea Party opposition.

Two facets of legislative capacity shape who is empowered to make decisions and may affect the likelihood that pockets of expertise will emerge. First, nearly everyone interviewed in Michigan believed term limits to be enormously consequential, resulting in legislators having little institutional or policy knowledge. There were no clear leaders on health policy that Republicans in the Michigan legislature could look to for guidance. The Michigan Speaker was only in his third year in elected office, and no one in leadership in either chamber had been in their role for very long. By contrast, the lack of term limits in Idaho means that on average, the leadership of the Idaho legislature has been in office for ten years. As a result of their relative longevity, legislators in Idaho have developed knowledge of their niche issues and of the legislative process as well as deep relationships.

Fifteen states place limits on how many terms their legislators are allowed to serve, generally restricting them to six to twelve years (Table 6.1). In some states, the clock resets if the legislator changes chambers or is out of power for a certain period. In other states, there are lifetime limits preventing the legislators from ever serving again (NCSL 2013). The term limit movement took off in the early 1990s, passing by directive initiative in twenty of the twenty-two states that voted for them, and being instituted by statute in two other states. Between 1997 and 2004, the state supreme

Table 6.1. TERM LIMITS IN STATE LEGISLATURES

		House		Senate	
State	Year Enacted	Limit	Year of Impact	Limit	Year of Impact
Maine	1993	8	1996	8	1996
California	1990	12[a]	1996	12[a]	1998
Colorado	1990	8	1998	8	1998
Arkansas	1992	6	1998	8	2000
Michigan	1992	6	1998	8	2002
Florida	1992	8	2000	8	2000
Ohio	1992	8	2000	8	2000
South Dakota	1992	8	2000	8	2000
Montana	1992	8	2000	8	2000
Arizona	1992	8	2000	8	2000
Missouri	1992	8	2002	8	2002
Oklahoma	1990	12[a]	2004	12[a]	2004
Nebraska	2000	n/a	n/a	8	2006
Louisiana	1995	12	2007	12	2007
Nevada	1996	12	2010	12	2010

[a] In California and Oklahoma, a legislator may serve a total of 12 years in the legislature during his or her lifetime. The total time may be split between the two chambers, or spent in its entirely in a single chamber. Before 2012, California's limits were identical to those in Arkansas: six years in the assembly and eight years in the senate.

courts in Massachusetts, Oregon, Washington, and Wyoming overturned their state's term limits, while the Idaho and Utah legislatures repealed theirs (Mooney 2009).

Advocates argue that term limits make legislators more responsive to their constituents, nontraditional candidates better situated to run, the seniority system weaker, and the relationship between legislators and special interests weaker, and that state spending would decrease as a result (Greenberg 1994, Masket and Lewis 2007, Basham 2011). The evidence supporting these arguments is mixed at best. Instead, studies show that under term limits, legislators are less beholden to constituents in their districts (Carey et al. 2006), in part because they are more likely to run for higher office (Powell 2000, Lazarus 2006). The number of bills introduced has spiked as legislators have less time to make their mark (Kousser 2004), resulting in increased state spending (Erler 2007). Under term limits, there are more lobbyists and they exert more influence in the legislative process (Mooney 2005). The power of legislative leaders has diminished (Apollonio and La Raja 2006), putting the executive branch in a stronger position relative to the legislature (Carey et al. 2006). Given all these consequences of legislative term limits, bipartisan negotiation and consensus building has been more difficult (Sarbaugh-Thompson et al. 2006).

Second, the amount of time a legislature stays in session varies from state to state and affects the ability of politicians to develop expertise (McDonough and McGrath 2001, Squire 2007, Burns et al. 2008). Most state legislatures only meet for part of the year. Thirty-nine states specify a limit on the length of their session, with seventeen of these having different limits in alternating years (NCSL 2013). Texas—the state with the second-highest population—has a legislature that only meets every other year. With the exception of Kentucky, Louisiana, and Virginia, states with different session lengths have the longer session in odd numbered years, resulting in shorter sessions during election years. Since Louisiana and Virginia hold their legislative elections in odd numbered years, the effect is the same. In states such as New Mexico, the legislature is restricted in alternating years to only considering bills amending the budget and is not allowed to consider bills on new policy such as creating a health insurance exchange.

Although longer sessions may increase the likelihood that legislators develop expertise, the fight over health insurance exchanges suggests that shorter sessions might ironically increase the influence of anyone who has expertise. The length of session, which is correlated to the amount legislators receive in salary, affects who can serve. Legislators need to wait until they retire or have a good day job to return to if they are in a state with short sessions. Approximately 2% of state legislators self-identify as working in insurance (Ehrenhalt 2015). They might have greater influence in the states with the least professionalized legislatures. The year-round legislative calendar therefore may compound the problem of inexperience and ignorance, limiting the amount of real-world experience legislators bring. Even the legislators themselves described bewilderment that such important health policy decisions were being made by people with so little health policy knowledge. The fact that staff support is more limited in the supposedly less professionalized states (NCLS 2009) might increase the degree to which they rely on colleagues they believe have developed expertise on an issue.

The general lack of expertise in the legislature on health policy gave some interest groups a greater role than they might have had otherwise. This seems to have amplified the ability of the Tea Party and conservative groups to shape the narrative. The role of interest groups was different in New Mexico, where there were not loud voices opposing the exchange. Legislators with the most expertise retired before the 2013 session, leaving a vacuum of knowledge about health policy in the legislature. This void was filled in part by people like Gail Evans of the Center on Law and Poverty, who legislators say was their chief negotiator in conversations with the governor. Governor Martinez had a point person, Matt Kennicott, coordinating the work being done by many people within the governor's office, multiple state agencies, and in the Office of Health Care Reform. Each of these people worked full-time and year-round. By contrast, legislators had minimal support and were in session only a few months per year. Consumer groups like the Center on Law and Poverty helped legislators make up the gap in expertise and attention. Interest groups aligned with the governor, such as the insurance industry, did not need to play the same role because the same need did not exist.

In addition to affecting the development of expertise, the timing of legislative sessions greatly shaped the contours of the debate in each state. The Mississippi legislature did not have an opportunity to weigh in on the exchange debate after its 2011 session because it did not meet again until well after Insurance Commissioner Chaney had begun planning. Similarly, the New Mexico legislature only had two 60-day windows to act between the ACA's passage in March 2010 and the beginning of open enrollment in October 2013. The first of these, in January through March 2011 was so early that the full intergovernmental context was not yet clear. This session also came immediately after Governor Martinez took office and before many people felt that she had her legs under her (Interviews 2013–2014). Had legislators been able to negotiate with her more fully before the start of the session, they might have chosen to advance a more modest bill that would have won her approval. After Governor Martinez's veto of SB 38 in 2011, the legislature did not have a serious opportunity to weigh in until the run-up to the 2013 session, leaving her in full control of the process until then. At that point the decision to run an exchange was too late, because there was not enough time to do everything necessary to avoid reliance on the federal government.

Federal leaders miscalculated the importance of the confluence of expertise and institutional capacity throughout the intergovernmental negotiation over health insurance exchanges. The Obama administration should have appreciated by mid-2012 that the timing of state legislative sessions worked against them (see Table 6.2). Of the states that had yet to create an exchange, only seven would still be in session after the Supreme Court released its ruling in *NFIB v. Sebelius*. Because the final level 2 establishment grant deadline was June 29, any state wanting to consider an exchange after that point would need to spend its own money. Even after the grant deadline was extended, governors in red states were unlikely to stick their neck out to create an exchange while the legislature was out of session until January or February 2013.

Table 6.2. LENGTH OF STATE LEGISLATIVE SESSIONS IN 2012

	Jan	Feb	Mar	Apr	May	Jun	Jul	Aug	Sep	Oct	Nov	Dec
Alabama												
Alaska												
Arizona												
Arkansas												
California												
Colorado												
Connecticut												
Delaware												
Florida												
Georgia												
Hawaii												
Idaho												
Illinois												
Indiana												
Iowa												
Kansas												
Kentucky												
Louisiana												
Maine												
Maryland												
Massachusetts												
Michigan												
Minnesota												
Mississippi												
Missouri												

Table 6.2. CONTINUED

	Jan	Feb	Mar	Apr	May	Jun	Jul	Aug	Sep	Oct	Nov	Dec
Montana												
Nebraska[a]												
Nevada												
New Hampshire												
New Jersey												
New Mexico												
New York												
North Carolina												
North Dakota												
Ohio												
Oklahoma												
Oregon												
Pennsylvania												
Rhode Island												
South Carolina												
South Dakota												
Tennessee												
Texas												
Utah												
Vermont												
Virginia												
Washington												
West Virginia												
Wisconsin												
Wyoming												

Note: States coded by partisan control: light shading = Fully Democratic, dark shading = Fully Republican, striped = Mixed

Vertical lines depict the Supreme Court decision announced June 28th and the election on November 6th

[a] Nebraska's legislature is officially non-partisan, but the state is led by a Republican governor

Source: NCSL 2012.

Leadership

The fourth insight from the states highlighted throughout this book is the importance of leadership. This is similar to the first point, which describes gubernatorial leadership as being particularly important. What I am saying here is more of a theoretical point, that two people facing similar environmental constraints and incentives may arrive at different conclusions and differ in their ability to build a coalition. This may seem obvious, but it is very difficult for political scientists to model differences in leadership capacity and judgment. Most examinations to date for why states have made certain decisions about the ACA use quantitative methods that abstract institutions such as the legislature and the governor to a single variable. This has value, but fails to capture the emotion, drama, and personalities behind these decisions.

For example, Phil Bryant made different decisions as governor than Haley Barbour said he would have made had he still been in office (Interview January 2014). Many Republicans in Idaho said they would have fought the exchange had they been governor instead of Butch Otter. Governor Otter was particularly effective at winning support for an exchange in Idaho. He made key strategic decisions such as putting his name on the legislation, having his chief of staff introduce the bills, and coordinating the stakeholder coalition through his office. Even this would not have the same effect if done by a different governor. Enough Republicans were wary of crossing Otter that they went along with him in a way that did not seem possible for governors elsewhere. Again, this might seem like stating the obvious, but the story of health insurance exchanges makes it clear that charisma, charm, personality, guts, and relationships matter tremendously in politics and in ways not easily built into quantitative statistical models.

WHAT SHOULD THE OBAMA ADMINISTRATION HAVE DONE DIFFERENTLY?

One reading of this book is that health insurance exchanges represent a major disappointment for the Obama administration. They tried to convince every state to create its own exchange, yet only 16 did. Approximately $1 billion was given to states that ultimately rejected control (Centers for Medicare and Medicaid Services [CMS] 2014). Many of the most supportive states, including Hawaii, Oregon, and Maryland, spent hundreds of millions of dollars trying to build websites that ultimately did not work.

Even Massachusetts—whose exchange served as the model for the ACA—struggled intensely during the first year of enrollment.

The challenges in these states may reflect the inability of government to manage large IT projects more than a specific failure by the Obama administration. A number of people interviewed said that one of the most important lessons from the exchanges is the challenge government has with managing vendors to do IT and other implementation activities (Interviews 2015–2016). This is a different question from the one I address of why so few states decided to create their own exchange—but they are closely intertwined. The administration spent a lot more energy and time trying to convince states to create an exchange than expected, complicating their planning for October 2013, when the first open enrollment period would begin. Many people at the state and federal level feel this contributed—along with not having been allocated any money to operate exchanges—to a disastrous rollout in October 2013, when Healthcare.gov tried to go live in many more states than it initially expected. They feel that key federal leaders were so focused on the intergovernmental politics that they did not hear—or did not sufficiently empower—people who were warning that the website would not be ready (Interviews 2014–2016).

The Obama administration repeatedly faced a catch-22 over how to deal with states. If it held firm to deadlines and expectations, opponents would accuse it of ignoring local needs and being too rigid. When deadlines were extended and flexibility was given, opponents pushed back further, stalling until after the Supreme Court ruling in June 2012 and the presidential election in November 2012. They saw the repeated extensions as evidence that the administration was bluffing and incapable of following through with its threats of preemption. But HHS feared that doing anything to prepare for the possibility that they would be running dozens of exchanges would undermine their efforts to convince states to comply. Many of the most dramatic moments highlighted in this book—such as the feud between Mississippi's commissioner and governor or the vote by the Michigan House Health Policy Committee—would not have happened had the Obama administration been firm on its deadlines, because states would have run out of time to make decisions.

This raises the question of what the Obama administration should have done differently in dealing with states. However, even with hindsight it is unclear whether it would have been better to hold firm to the deadlines. The problems with preparing for exchanges may have been more fundamental than this. In the wake of the troubled rollout of the federal exchange in the fall of 2013, the *Washington Post* published a memo Harvard economist

David Cutler (2010) had written three years earlier warning that the ACA's implementation was off track. He argued that HHS was a deeply flawed organization and that a separate entity should be created to bring together government and industry leaders to oversee implementation.

Michael Doonan (2013) similarly called for the creation of a "Center for State-Based Health Exchanges" to work closely with a wide variety of stakeholders to "foster collaboration, align incentives, share information, and document and publicize successes." These proposals likely would have made the Obama administration's oversight more efficient and improved planning of the federal exchange, potentially avoiding the disastrous early days of open enrollment. But this would not necessarily have influenced more states to decide to create their own exchange.

The Obama administration, along with the reporters and academics writing about this negotiation, should have better appreciated the complexities of state politics in their outreach, including the importance of legislators and pockets of expertise. Regular channels were developed by federal leaders for constant communication with the governor's office and/or a designated agency in each state. By definition of HHS's rules, no exchange could be created without a governor's approval. However, Michigan and Mississippi illustrate that gubernatorial support was not enough.

HHS took phone calls from legislators, but did not seem to have a strategy to reach out to them directly. This reinforced the asymmetry in expertise between bureaucrats and most legislators, putting pressure on agency officials to "educate" the politicians. At the same time, federal officials connecting directly with legislators would have created problems with state executive branch leaders, who would view this as meddling. It likely was not worth the risk for HHS that they would lose a governor. This is a tough situation to navigate for federal officials trying to encourage state cooperation.

Complicating the picture further is the observation by a number of people involved that the different parts of the federal government were not always on the same page (Interviews 2011–2016). The Center for Consumer Information and Insurance Oversight (CCIIO) within the Department of Health and Human Services was the primary contact for most state leaders working on creating an exchange. But many of the most important decisions were made by the White House. The denial of Insurance Commissioner Mike Chaney's exchange proposal in Mississippi suggests that strong connections between legislators and CCIIO might not be enough because White House officials might make different decisions anyway.

DOES IT MATTER?

This book is about how states decided what type of exchange to establish, including whether to run their own exchange or default to the federal government. It is worth reflecting on whether this choice matters. One way to look at this is to examine how well states did at signing people up for insurance. Some of the most resistant states were in the top ten in terms of the percentage of eligible people who enrolled in the first year, with Florida at fourth, Michigan at sixth, Maine at eighth, and North Carolina at ninth. Idaho and Michigan took divergent paths on the question of whether or not to create an exchange, yet signed up essentially the exact same proportion of eligible residents (37.7% in Idaho vs. 37.6% in Michigan). Eight states that chose to run their own exchange finished below the national average, including four of the worse ten (KFF 2014c). Similar patterns were seen in subsequent years.

Buried in these numbers are some reasons why high enrollment may still be easier to achieve for states that chose to run their own exchange. Looking beyond the top 10, Blumberg, Buettgens, and Holahan (2015) found that state-based marketplaces as a whole enrolled 76% of the projected population in the first year compared to 54% in states with a federally facilitated marketplace (note the distinction between eligible population and projected population). One reason may be that the ACA allows the federal government to give state-based exchanges larger grants to help with enrollment and consumer outreach. Community organizations in the thirty-four states that rejected control received a combined total of $67 million for the first year of enrollment, for an average of less than $2 million per state. By contrast, California and Maryland each spent $37 million and $24 million on outreach for the same period (Jost 2013).

Enroll America, an organization run by former Obama operatives, ran aggressive enrollment campaigns in some of the states that rejected control of an exchange. As in a political campaign gearing up for an election, they hired people to go door to door signing people up for coverage. They targeted states with large numbers of uninsured people, including some that had voted for President Obama in recent elections such as Florida and Michigan (Somashekhar 2013). This may help explain why these states finished in the top ten of enrollment in 2014, although this did little outside states targeted by Enroll America and it is uncertain whether this is sustainable in the long term.

Enrollment in and of itself is not the only way an insurance exchange should be judged. State-based exchanges are better able to innovate and tailor their efforts. They can develop more stringent requirements for qualified health plans. States with their own exchange may have more robust competition because insurers are more willing to participate. Interviewees in some states—such as Mississippi—say that insurers who chose to not sell plans in the federal exchange likely would have participated had the state been in charge (Interviews 2014–2015). State exchanges also have lower user fees than the federal exchange and are better positioned to solve problems as they arise. Leaders in Idaho describe a night and day difference between the experience of fully running their own exchange in 2015 compared to relying on the federal website in 2014. There was previously very little they could do to help consumers who had mistakenly lost benefits or had some other problems. Once the state took over they were able to look up information in their own systems and quickly resolve any problems (Interviews 2014–2016).

King v. Burwell

The Supreme Court's decision in November 2014 to consider *King v. Burwell* dramatically increased the stakes of the fight over health insurance exchanges and would have provided a definitive answer to the question of whether it mattered who runs an exchange. The case was the culmination of the second major line of attack on Obamacare after the Supreme Court ruling and reelection of President Obama in 2012. The argument hinged on the interpretation of four words in the law. The ACA states that people can receive tax credits if they buy insurance through an exchange "established by the state." Should the administration interpret this to literally mean that no consumer is allowed to receive financial assistance from the federal government if they live in a state that refused to create an exchange?

Many experts dismissed the case as lacking merit. Jeffrey Toobin (2015) described it as "a shameful and cynical exercise which illustrated the debasement of the contemporary legal movement." Nicholas Bagley (2015) compared opponents to Amelia Bedelia, the character in children's books who misunderstands everything by taking instructions too literally. He wrote that Scalia and others were "transform[ing] statutory interpretation into a game of gotcha, where slipshod drafting is an excuse to ignore persuasive clues about what Congress meant to communicate." An amicus brief filed by health policy scholars – which I signed - traced the legislative history of insurance exchanges to suggest that these four words should be read in a broader context such that Congress would not intend to restrict subsidies to people in state-based exchanges (Jost et al. 2015).

By making it to the Supreme Court's docket, however, the case had major potential to upend a core element of the ACA. A ruling for the plaintiffs would have triggered a series of events estimated to result in declines of health insurance coverage for 9.6 million people. Only the sickest would keep their insurance, resulting in significantly more expensive risk pools. Insurers would therefore raise rates for everyone, including people not on the exchange, leading to estimated increases in premiums of as high as 47% (Saltzman and Eibner 2015).

Supreme Court rules requiring four justices to want to hear a case suggested that at least that many had serious doubt about the administration's interpretation (Bagley, Jones, and Jost 2015). Supporters of the law initially dismissed the implications of the law, since states would face so much pressure if the plaintiffs won that they would quickly move to establish an exchange, which legally allowed people to receive subsidies. Bagley, Jones, and Jost (2015) were not so optimistic, since "an exchange is not just a website and setting up one requires a sizeable investment of time and resources." States would face enormously complicated questions about how to establish authority under tight time pressures and how to develop all the functionality of an exchange in a matter of months when other states struggled to do so over four years. How would state leaders pay for all this, since exchanges were supposed to be financially self-sufficient by 2015 and given that HHS no longer had authority to give out grants for exchange development (Bagley and Jones 2015)?

Convincing these states to move quickly would have been difficult, especially since these thirty-four states were by definition the most strongly opposed to an exchange. Even if state leaders were willing to cooperate, intense time pressures would have made this difficult. The HHS regulations required that states wanting to establish an exchange needed to apply for conditional approval six and a half months before going live. The next enrollment period was scheduled to begin on November 15, less than five months after the Court was expected to rule. Further compounding the challenge was the reality that only eight of the thirty-four affected states would have legislative sessions in the latter half of 2014 (Bagley, Jones, and Jost 2015).

Leaders in these states were in a very difficult position during the months they spent in limbo. Opponents were reluctant to do anything that would align them with the Obama administration. Supporters worried that developing contingency plans would undermine their position that the lawsuit lacked merit, since it showed they worried the government would lose. The Obama administration repeatedly said it was so confident it would win that it was doing nothing to prepare for the possibility that it would not.

State leaders also anticipated that Congress and the administration would react to the ruling, thereby changing the nature of the options available to states. Any planning prior to the ruling would therefore be a waste of time. Meanwhile, state-level Republicans worried they would be blamed if people lost their coverage (Jones et al. 2015).

Drama built as the end of the Court's session drew near in late June 2015. Congressional Republicans wrote op-eds saying that they had plans under development which would protect anyone from losing coverage (Hatch, Alexander, and Barasso 2015). Conservatives hoped these would convince any undecided members of the Supreme Court that the administration was exaggerating its predictions about what was at stake. Legislation was introduced in both the House and Senate, including a bill cosponsored by Senate Majority Leader Mitch McConnell (S.1016 2015). However, there was little indication that Republicans would be able to unite behind a single post-King plan (Klein 2015).

State leaders were unsure of how to prepare. A confidential meeting was convened by the Millbank Memorial Fund in June 2015 in which leaders from New Mexico and Idaho, along with Nevada who had gone a similar route when their eligibility system had not worked, shared their experiences with advisors to governors and state agency heads such as insurance commissioners and secretaries of health from nearly twenty states (Koller 2015). This "secret huddle" at an O'Hare Airport hotel gave states a chance to compare notes on their options with regard to *King v. Burwell* (Radnofsky and Armour 2015). Delaware and Pennsylvania subsequently submitted proposals to become a state-based exchange, making sure that their applications were in and they received conditional approval by June 15 (Pradhan 2015). This was a protective measure to satisfy the requirement that applications be received six and a half months before a new exchange went live. A bill introduced in New Hampshire was nicknamed "the magic wand," because it would have changed the legal status while doing nothing else different (Jones et al. 2015). This was also called the "dub thee" option, as in the legislature would now be saying "I dub thee to be a state exchange" even though nothing changes (Interviews 2015). It is not clear whether this would have passed legal muster, but it would have bought the state time to keep residents covered.

On June 25 the Supreme Court announced its 6–3 ruling in favor of the Obama administration. Chief Justice John Roberts and Anthony Kennedy joined the four liberals on the court, with Roberts writing the opinion. He explained that the law should be read so that "state exchanges and federal exchanges are equivalent—they meet the same requirements, perform the same functions, and serve the same purposes." He concluded, "it is implausible that Congress meant the Act to operate" in a way that restricted tax credits, since "Congress passed the Affordable Care Act to improve health insurance markets, not to destroy them. If at all possible, we must interpret the Act in a way that is consistent with the former and avoids the latter" (*King v. Burwell* 2015).

Justice Antonin Scalia was livid. He called the decision "pure applesauce" and "interpretative jiggery-pokery" because of its "somersaults of statutory interpretation." He chastised Roberts and the rest of the majority for lacking shame and suggested "we should start calling this law SCOTUScare" since the Court saved the law twice (*King v. Burwell* 2015).

The Affordable Care Act survived *King v. Burwell*. However, this still did not mean the law was invincible. More lawsuits were filed, including by the House of Representatives over the Obama administration's use of funds to implement an aspect of the law despite no clear appropriation by Congress. In December 2015 the US Senate finally voted to repeal the ACA, something the House had already done more than fifty times. President Obama vetoed the bill in January 2016. Donald Trump went on to win the presidency in 2016 on a platform of repealing Obamacare. As of this writing it is unclear whether he and Congressional Republicans will follow through with their threats.

LOOKING FORWARD

The Supreme Court's ruling in 2015 did not end fighting over the ACA, but did mean that states could continue as they were with respect to health insurance exchanges and that people with eligible incomes could receive federal subsidies to purchase insurance. Consumers in states refusing to participate could continue to rely on the national website healthcare.gov. States wanting more control would continue to move in this direction.

I now turn to two final questions: First, assuming the law survives existential threats such as the possibility of repeal or further litigation, what is the future of health insurance exchanges? Second, what can we learn from this episode about the future of health reform and US federalism more broadly?

The Future of Health Insurance Exchanges

It is very difficult to make predictions about the future of health reform from the vantage point of early 2017. A Republican-led Congress has built incredibly high expectations that it will work with President Donald Trump to repeal major components of the ACA and has already passed legislation in the House. But let us assume for a moment that they do not make any changes or that Hillary Clinton had won the election. Would more states have decided to reclaim control over their exchange from the federal government or had a new status quo emerged in which states are locked into the decision they made prior to 2014? As described earlier, this is fundamentally different from the similar question of whether more states will expand Medicaid. The loss of money for the state budget and the number of people going without insurance coverage make it likely that most states will ultimately accept the Medicaid expansion. States now have very little to gain for all the work that would be required by choosing to take control of their exchange. The requirement for state exchanges to be financially self-sustaining is a high hurdle, particularly now that states can no longer receive federal grants. It is unlikely that very many, if any, will decide to switch to a state-based exchange.

The dynamic between states and the federal government changed after the exchanges went live in 2014. A subtle shift took place, and was crystallized with the ruling in *King v. Burwell*, in which the federal government is no longer desperate for states to step up. Healthcare.gov had a disastrous beginning but is functional and continually improving. Federal call centers are in place, and enrollment targets are consistently met. Changing arrangements with states might be more complicated at this point than it would be helpful.

Two states have tried to build their own websites since 2014: Idaho and New Mexico. Idaho's experience demonstrates that a motivated state could move from using healthcare.gov to developing its own. After using the federal website in 2014, the state was able to create its own site in time for the 2015 enrollment. But its experience was so unique that it might serve more as a warning than a model for other states interested in a similar evolution. It had a very different starting point than any other state considering this approach going forward. Although it relied on the federal website the first year, the law passed in March 2013 meant that Idaho was officially designated a state-based exchange. It had an active board of directors, a respected executive director, and it insisted on retaining control of regulatory decisions. It was able to apply for the large level 2 establishment grant for state-based exchanges before the deadlines passed.

Leaders in Idaho described the federal government as a subcontractor, while at the same time acknowledging the confusing dynamic in which the federal government was also the ultimate authority. Idaho was able to migrate from healthcare.gov to its own website largely because the state had already invested significant resources in upgrading its Medicaid eligibility systems. This technology could be leveraged as a front door through which people could access the exchange. States that had not already made these changes would likely have a hard time affording a new site, especially in the absence of federal grants. The exchange also creatively partnered with insurance agents and brokers to save the state money by doing advertising and promotion on behalf of the exchange. The relationship with agents and brokers is much more adversarial in other states, making this an unlikely option.

New Mexico's experience after 2014 epitomized the new dynamic between states and the federal government and the challenge that other states could face. Their exchange legislation was passed in March 2013 on the same day as Idaho's. The newly formed board quickly realized it was too late to develop their own technology in time for the beginning of open enrollment that October. Like Idaho, they decided to rely on the federal website for the first year while making plans to build their own website in time for the 2015 enrollment period.

In mid-2014 the board hired Amy Dowd as its executive director, the person who previously led Idaho's exchange. The board decided that the state's website would not be ready for 2015 and that it would be better to wait one more year than to rush toward a disastrous rollout. As the final deadline for a federal level 2 establishment grant approached in November 2014, the state submitted an application requesting $97.9 million to finish its website. The Obama administration did not approve the proposal. Their rejection specifically cited and rebutted the sharply worded letters that Governor Susana Martinez submitted with the application criticizing the Obama administration for what she considered new requirements that were onerous and difficult to achieve (Martinez 2014b). Without these funds, the state lacked the ability to develop its own technology and would continue to rely on the federal website while still ostensibly being a state-based insurance exchange. People on either side of the debate either criticize Governor Martinez for how she handled this or the Obama administration for their decision.

Regardless of whose version of the story is accurate, this was the first time the Obama administration had rejected a state's exchange grant application during the ACA's implementation. Up until this point, states had always received money every time they submitted an exchange grant. The federal government had been a virtually blank check. The rejected grant application made it clear that this was no longer true.

Plans for transitioning to state-run exchanges in Delaware and Pennsylvania were immediately abandoned once the Supreme Court ruled with the Obama administration in *King v. Burwell*. States like the idea of having user fees for their consumers below the federal level of 3.5%, but local control was not worth the work after the disaster of *King v. Burwell* had been adverted. There is little reason to think that other states will come to a different conclusion and will decide to move to a state-based exchange.

States could consider following the lead of New Mexico and Nevada by retaining control of decision-making but using the federal website for enrollment. However, the situation has changed in these states in ways that make this model less tenable. The federal government used to allow states to use the website rent-free, but will now be charging a fee (Interview July 2016). Unless something changes, it is unlikely that more states will take this approach—or any other—to transition from a federal exchange to one that is state operated.

If there is any movement, it will likely be in the direction of states giving up and ceding some control back to the federal government. Small states like Rhode Island are in a difficult position to fulfill the requirement that all exchanges be self-sustaining. One state has already undone its decision to run an exchange. Kentucky Governor Steve Beshear established Kynect in July 2012 after his legislature failed to act. This made Kentucky the only state in the south to operate its own exchange. He did the same with Medicaid expansion. The implementation of both programs went very well and was considered a national model. President Obama even invited Governor Beshear to the State of the Union and praised his leadership. Approximately 425,000 gained coverage in Kentucky as a result of the ACA, bringing the uninsured rate down from 14% in 2013 to 6% in 2015 (Barnett and Vornovitsky 2016). This is a stunning decrease in such a short period of time.

These gains would likely have been maintained or even improved had Kentuckyians elected Democrat Jack Conway as their next governor. Instead, they voted for Matt Bevin, whose campaign platform consisted of getting rid of Obamacare in Kentucky (Jones 2015). Reminiscent of the question "What's the Matter with Kansas," (Bartels 2006) people in the parts of the state that benefited the most from the ACA voted overwhelmingly for Bevin. Polling shows that 63% of Kentuckyians have a favorable view of Medicaid and 72% would rather keep the program rather than take away insurance from people (Hamel, Norton, and Brodie 2015). They may not have understood that getting rid of Obamacare would jeopardize their insurance, not realizing that Kynect is the state's version of the ACA.

Kentucky's experience is a good test for the question of whether it mattered if a state runs its own exchange. Eligible people will continue to receive federal tax credits through healthcare.gov. However, the state's website was a one-stop portal for multiple programs such as Medicaid, KCHIP, WIC, and SNAP. The decision to undo the state's exchange may jeopardize assistance through all of these programs. As early as September 2016—well before any benefits would be affected by changes made by Governor Bevin—leaders of local health departments said they were already seeing an increase in utilization from people who were concerned they were about to lose insurance (Interviews September 2016). Former Governor Steve Beshear is frustrated and disappointed, saying that "to knowingly jeopardize the health care of thousands of families in Kentucky is incomprehensible and irresponsible" (Yetter 2016).

Other state-based exchanges are likely not as vulnerable, because other than New York and Rhode Island—two states unlikely to see a major shift in attitude from leadership about the ACA—they were created by legislation rather than executive order. In other words, the same institutional forces that made it hard to pass a law creating an exchange would make it difficult to pass a law undoing an exchange.

The Future of Health Reform

The 2016 election makes the previous paragraphs more of a thought exercise than an analysis on what is likely to happen. But the fight over health insurance exchanges detailed in this book provides important insights for future attempts at reform, whether these reforms are focused on repealing the ACA or sometime further down the road expanding coverage further. Federalism is likely to be an appealing solution to the political challenge of winning sufficient consensus in Congress to pass anything. Many Republican proposals to dismantle Barack Obama's signature reform focus on giving states significant choices, in some cases even to keep major ACA programs. Liberal states might find that pushing for increased flexibility from the Trump administration will be the best way to mitigate the damages. If the ACA is repealed, the next Democratic president and Congress will face enormous pressure to pass new health reform restoring coverage expansions.

Given the complexities of trying to simultaneously move forward on fifty fronts, should the lesson from this episode be that supporters of health reform or other broad initiatives avoid federalism and focus on national solutions? Not necessarily. For one, this is not a fair question, since the ACA would not have passed absent a large role for states. Reformers likely would rather struggle through a complex implementation than have no reform at all.

There are many other examples of policies in which the federal government has convinced states to participate despite partisan tension, including two major health insurance programs: Medicaid and the Children's Health Insurance Program (CHIP) (Grogan and Rigby 2009). Every state now administers both programs and few would likely seriously consider backing out. The lawsuit that led to the ACA case before the Supreme Court in 2012 was based on state leaders protesting coercive threats that would have eliminated their Medicaid programs. When CHIP was up for reauthorization in 2015, 80% of governors wrote letters calling on Congress to continue the program, including many Republicans who opposed the ACA (Oberlander and Jones 2015). But the fight over insurance exchanges illustrates that the federal government does not have an unlimited ability to compel states to do what it wants. It should be modest and realistic in its expectations when asking states to play a prominent role in health and in other policy domains such as education or environmental reform.

The federal government's leverage in negotiating with states is affected by the nature of the policy in question. The contrast with Medicaid and CHIP reveals an important characteristic of the negotiation over exchanges. When push came to shove, the incentives to take the initiative on building an exchange—the promise of money and the threat of preemption—were not as strong as expected. Yes there were programmatic advantages of local control such as the potential for better coordination with Medicaid eligibility systems and the ability to determine whether their exchange would be a highly regulated active purchaser or a looser clearinghouse. There were also political reasons for states to want local control as well, since this was the preference of their major interest groups.

But as Béland, Rocco, and Waddan (2016) point out, exchanges were particularly susceptible to the politics of dissent because their high level of institutional fragmentation was combined with a relatively high level of public salience, low level of public support, and weak policy legacies. Unlike with the Medicaid expansion, in which money would flow into state budgets and into the hands of key interest groups, state flexibility over the exchanges brought weak fiscal incentives. Medicaid money would not come if states did not opt in to the expansion. Exchange money would come regardless of what the state did. In addition, states benefited very little from the money they received to establish exchanges. These federal grants simply covered the expense of hiring IT vendors, consultants, or additional staff to work under terms dictated by HHS. Many state leaders came to see their role in the exchange as doing the Obama administration's dirty work without getting much in return.

The threat of a federal takeover came to be viewed as a safety net. There was very little risk for a governor or legislator to oppose an exchange. Every eligible person in their state would still receive the subsidies to make insurance more affordable, regardless of whether it was through a state-based or federally run exchange. By contrast, a state refusing to expand Medicaid was foregoing millions of dollars and denying insurance coverage to large numbers of people. By dragging their feet for so long on the exchange, opponents hoped they were increasing the likelihood that it would fail and Obamacare would collapse. If that happened, the Obama administration would take the blame, not state leaders for standing up to the president. If the program was successful and popular, state leaders believed they might still be able to convince voters that they deserved credit.

Supporters of even more comprehensive health reform should recognize the challenges that reliance on federalism brings. Pursuing a national strategy does not ensure that all of these challenges will be avoided, but does take away an opportunity for perpetuating postenactment obstructionism. Even so, the ACA strengthens the role that states play in the governance and financing of healthcare in the United States. The realities of path dependence are such that it will be very difficult for any substantial health reforms to not take this into account and include at least some room for state adaptation.

State-level resistance to health insurance exchanges was stunning and unexpected, epitomizing the messiness of intergovernmental politics. The ability of exchange legislation to pass in Idaho—one of the most conservative states in the country—makes it clear that no state was destined to make the choice it did. Every state was up for grabs. The story of the ACA and the health insurance exchanges is far from over. Supporters will continue to work on strengthening the reform just as opponents will continue to undo it.

This is just one of the many marble cakes created by ever-evolving and overlapping boundaries between states and the federal government. One of the lasting consequences of this episode may be an increased confidence among state leaders to resist federal policy it does not like. As with health insurance exchanges, we can expect states will be in a difficult position of navigating internal battles at the same time as trying to influence national policy. A major lesson for federal and state reformers is that the process of determining who in a state makes decisions is not always straightforward and can be as contentious as debates over which policies to adopt.

APPENDIX A

Timeline of Key Events in Mississippi

PRE-AFFORDABLE CARE ACT

- 2007: Governor Haley Barbour (R) publicly supports creating an exchange.
- 2008: Two bills to create an exchange were introduced in the Senate, one by Democrat Hob Bryan and one by Republican Eugene Clark. Clark's bill passed the Senate unanimously but was never voted on in the House.
- 2009: Governor Barbour mentions the exchange in his state of the state speech. Once again, a Republican bill passed with bipartisan support in the Senate but did not receive a vote in the House.
- 2009: The legislature amends the statute governing the Mississippi Comprehensive Health Insurance Risk Pool Association (MCHIRPA) to expand the insurance commissioner's authority over other state and federal insurance programs.

2010

- March 23: Affordable Care Act (ACA) is signed into law by President Obama.
- September 30: Insurance Department receives a $1 million planning grant.
- November: Mississippi is one of the few states that does not hold legislative elections in even numbered years. However, by the start of the next legislative session, enough Senate Democrats switched parties to give Republicans control of the chamber.

2011

- January–March: Four exchange bills were introduced, three in the House and one in the Senate. Each chamber approved a bill, though a conference committee could not agree on a compromise and no legislation was enacted.
- August 12: HHS awards the Insurance Department with a $20 million level 1 establishment grant. The application outlined plans to use MCHIRPA to create an exchange without legislative approval.
- November 8: Phil Bryant (R) is elected governor. Republicans won full control of both chambers for the first time since Reconstruction in the nineteenth century. Bryant did not focus on the ACA on the campaign trail, but indicated he would continue to support an exchange.

2012

- January: Insurance Department begins holding meetings of an exchange advisory board comprising industry leaders and other stakeholders.
- June 28: The US Supreme Court announces its ruling upholding the ACA and making the Medicaid expansion optional.
- July 11: Tea Party leaders speak for the first time at a meeting of the exchange advisory board. The Tea Party continued to mobilize, subsequently attending meetings of the Personnel Review Board and blocking contracts with exchange vendors.
- November 6: Barack Obama is reelected president. Insurance Commissioner Mike Chaney responds by saying he is ready to submit the state's blueprint once he discusses it with the governor.
- November 12: Governor Bryant and Commissioner Chaney meet at the Governor's Mansion, with Bryant saying he will oppose the application and Chaney saying he will submit it anyway. As an independently elected official himself, Chaney believed he did not need the governor's approval.
- November 26: Governor Bryant writes the Department of Health and Human Services (HHS) Secretary Kathleen Sebelius to oppose the application submitted by Commissioner Chaney.

2013

- January 15: Mississippi Attorney General Jim Hood (D) issues a report agreeing with Commissioner Chaney that Governor Bryant's approval is not needed.

- January 18: Governor Bryant writes Secretary Sebelius another letter, this time criticizing Attorney General Hood's report and saying that he would instruct the Mississippi Division of Medicaid not to cooperate with an exchange established by Commissioner Chaney.
- February 7: HHS rejects the Insurance Department's exchange application.
- July 1: Deadline by which Medicaid needed to be renewed. Democrats tried to use this moment as leverage to push Republicans to support expansion. A special session was called in which Medicaid was renewed but not expanded.
- October 1: On the same day that open enrollment begins, HHS approves a plan submitted by Commissioner Chaney for the state to run the small business exchange while the federal government retains control of the individual exchange.

APPENDIX B

Timeline of Key Events in Michigan

2010

- March 23: ACA signed into law by President Obama. Michigan Attorney General Mike Cox (R) joins multistate lawsuit challenging the law's constitutionality.
- March 31: Governor Jennifer Granholm (D) creates the Health Insurance Reform Coordinating Council to oversee the ACA's implementation.
- September 30: The Department of Community Health (DCH) is awarded $1 million by the federal government for exchange planning.
- November 2: Rick Snyder (R) elected governor. Republicans win control of the House and win seats in the Senate. Republicans win their largest majorities since the early 1950s.
- December 2: The Coordinating Council releases its reporting recommending the state run its own exchange.

2011

- January 1: Rick Snyder (R) sworn in as governor.
- February–June: Public sector consultants tasked with leading work groups to solicit input from stakeholders. The final report was released June 17 and recommends Michigan develop its own clearinghouse exchange as a quasi-governmental organization.
- September 14: Governor Snyder releases a "special message on health," calling for the legislature to pass legislation creating an exchange by Thanksgiving.

- November 10: Senate passes SB 693 to create an exchange by a vote of 25–12.
- November 14: US Supreme Court announces it will consider the cases challenging the ACA's constitutionality.
- November 29: Department of Licensing and Regulatory Affairs (LARA) awarded $9.9-million level 1 establishment grant.
- December 13: House passes supplemental funding bill without authorizing LARA to spend its grant.

2012

- January 19: House Health Policy Committee holds its tenth hearing on the exchange without taking a vote. Thirty-one people testified at this meeting lasting more than three hours.
- June 28: US Supreme Court announces ruling upholding the ACA but making the Medicaid expansion optional; House Speaker Jase Bolger (R) and Committee Chair Gail Haines (R) continue to resist exchange.
- November 6: Barack Obama reelected President. Republican majority in the House reduced; House Speaker Jase Bolger (R) and Committee Chair Gail Haines (R) publicly support an exchange for the first time.
- November 15: Obama administration extends the deadline by which states need to decide.
- November 29: House Health Policy Committee vote 9–5 against an exchange bill that was tie-barred to an abortion bill. Four Democrats abstained or did not show up. One Republican did not vote.

2013

- January 17: LARA awarded $31 million level 1 establishment grant.
- January 22: Governor Snyder submits letter to HHS declaring plans to create a partnership exchange.
- February 28: House votes 78–31 to approve supplemental funding bill authorizing LARA to spend the $31-million level 1 establishment grant.
- March 5: HHS gives conditional approval of Michigan's partnership blueprint. The Senate never took a vote on the supplemental funding bill, effectively blocking the grant and preventing the state from doing the work required to operate a partnership exchange.
- September 16: Governor Snyder signs legislation expanding Medicaid.
- October 1: Open enrollment begins, Michigan is part of the federal exchange.

APPENDIX C

Timeline of Key Events in Idaho

2010

- March 17: Governor Otter signs the Idaho Health Freedom Act, banning public officials from playing any role in enforcing federal insurance mandates.
- March 23: ACA passes and Idaho Attorney General Lawrence Wasden joins the lawsuit.
- September 30: The Department of Insurance receives $1-million exchange planning grant.
- November 2: Governor Otter reelected and Republican majorities strengthened in both chambers.
- December: Governor Otter creates the Idaho Health Care Council to solicit stakeholder input.

2011

- February 16: Nullification bill HB 117 passed by the House 49–20.
- February 25: HB 117 defeated by the Senate State Affairs Committee on a voice vote.
- March 16: Senate approves funding of the exchange grant by a vote of 20-15. The House never voted, effectively blocking this grant from being spent.
- April 20: Governor Otter vetoes another nullification bill, which had been passed by the House (50–17) and the Senate (24–11). On the same

day as this veto, Governor Otter signs an executive order blocking state agencies from implementing the ACA, with the only exception being exchange planning.

2012

- January–March: No exchange legislation introduce in the 2012 legislative session.
- May 15: Republican primary elections reveal divisions within the House Republican caucus. House Speaker Lawrence Denney takes the unprecedented step of using his PAC money against incumbent Republicans.
- November 6: Barack Obama is reelected president. More than one-third of the legislature would be new in 2013 as a result of redistricting and retirements.
- November 15: HHS extends exchange deadline, giving Idaho a chance to reconsider.
- December 5: Scott Bedke becomes House Speaker after a summer-long campaign to oust Denney.
- December: Governor Otter announces support for a state-based exchange.

2013

- February 7: Exchange legislation (SB 1142) passes the Senate Commerce and Human Resources Committee 8–1 after two days of intense meetings.
- February 13: Sixteen House freshmen announce support for an exchange if more oversight is given to the legislature.
- February 21: Senate passes the original exchange bill 23–12 after a seven-hour debate.
- March 6: An alternative exchange bill (HB 248) passes the House Health and Welfare Committee on a voice vote.
- March 13: HB 248 passes 41–29 on the House floor.
- March 19: Senate Commerce and Human Resources Committees approves HB 248.
- March 21: Senate passes HB 248 by a vote of 23–12.
- March 28: Governor Otter signs the legislation creating a state-based exchange.

- April 10: Governor Otter appoints the nineteen-member board of directors without needing Senate confirmation because the legislative session had ended for the year. One of the first decisions made by the board was for Idaho to use the federal website for its exchange for in 2014.
- October 1: Open enrollment begins. Many Idahoans are confused about whether their state is operating its own exchange.

APPENDIX D

Timeline of Key Events in New Mexico

PRE-AFFORDABLE CARE ACT

- 2007–2008: The first exchange bills were introduced, largely at the urging of J. R. Damron, a radiologist who had been the Republican nominee for governor in 2006. Neither bill advanced, as Democrats controlling the legislature hoped for a more comprehensive reform.

2010

- July 1: Task force convened by Governor Richardson recommends New Mexico retain control of its exchange. Richardson creates the New Mexico Office of Health Care Reform to oversee implementation.
- November 2: Republican Susana Martinez is elected governor.
- December 27: Richardson's Office of Health Care Reform prepares a transition plan for the incoming Martinez administration. It includes a recommendation to pass legislation in the 2011 session to create a quasi-governmental exchange with active purchaser powers.

2011

- March 2: SB 38, one of the four exchange bills introduced that session, passes the Senate.
- March 19: SB 38 passes the House. The vote was very close, with Speaker Ben Luján calling the vote after midnight at the precise moment when there were just enough supporters in the chamber to ensure passage.

- April 8: Governor Martinez vetoes SB 38. She is not opposed to creating an exchange but would prefer a clearinghouse model in which insurers are allowed on the board. Her office created an exchange by executive order within the Health Insurance Alliance.
- August: Dan Derksen is appointed to lead the Office of Health Care Reform. He immediately announces plans to apply for a level 1 establishment grant before the September 30 deadline, as well as to apply for a level 2 grant by the following March. This implies formal authority would be received by then, most likely by executive order.
- September 30: Derksen submits a level 1 grant application requesting $34 million, including a letter from Governor Martinez saying she is "pleased to endorse" the proposal, which would create an exchange through the Alliance.

2012

- January–February: No exchange bills are considered during the legislative session because in even-numbered years, the legislature is only allowed to consider bills reacting to a special message from the governor or relating directly to the budget.
- March: Dan Derksen suddenly resigns due to opposition from Governor Martinez's advisors. The level 2 grant application was nearly ready but was never submitted.
- July 9: The legislature's Interim Health and Human Services Committee begins holding monthly meetings and discusses the exchange more than any other issue.
- September 11: Assistant Attorney General Mark Reynolds issues an opinion that Governor Martinez does not have authority to create an exchange by executive order since she vetoed similar legislation in the past. Her office backed down after Democrats threatened to sue.
- November 27: The Interim Committee endorses legislation create a clearinghouse exchange through the Alliance.

2013

- January: Governor Martinez announces support for expanding Medicaid. Four exchange bills are introduced, with regular negotiations between the governor's office and consumer advocates working with legislative Democrats.

- February 28: A bill to create an active purchaser exchange is defeated in the House, 30–39.
- March 15: A bill to create a clearinghouse exchange allowing insurers to serve on the board passes through multiple committees and both chambers in a single week once compromise was reached.
- March 28: Governor Martinez signs exchange legislation.
- April 29: The board of directors holds its first meeting, realizing there is not enough time to create an exchange before open enrollment begins.
- July: HHS grants conditional approval for New Mexico to run the SHOP exchange while still giving up control of the individual exchange for the first year.

NOTES

CHAPTER 1

1. To help states make these decisions and plan for the creation of an exchange, the federal government awarded four types of noncompetitive grants: (1) a planning grant of approximately $1 million; (2) an innovator grant ranging from $6 million to $54.5 million for a handful of states to take the lead in developing the IT infrastructure necessary to build an exchange; (3) level 1 establishment grants available on a quarterly basis; and (4) a level 2 establishment grant intended to carry exchanges to 2015, when they were to be self-sustaining. By February 2013, when most states had made their decision, 36 states and the District of Columbia had received average of about $37 million in level 1 establishment grants. One year later, when insurance exchanges were supposed to be operational, 15 states had received a total of $2.6 billion in level 2 grants, averaging $171 million per state (KFF 2014a).
2. This number includes Lincoln Chafee, who had been a Republican US Senator, was an independent as governor, but later ran for president as a Democrat.
3. Democrats had majorities in 28 of 44 legislative chambers in these states, and shared control of the Oregon House with Republicans. Roll call data was compiled from the legislative website of each state.
4. State Refor(u)m is a project funded by the Robert Wood Johnson Foundation and led by the National Academy for State Health Policy (NASHP). The document library can be found at www.statereforum.org

CHAPTER 3

1. Governor Snyder also announced his plan to lose 10 pounds in the coming year. By October 24 he had so far lost 6 pounds (AP 2011a). When pushed the following year whether he had met the goal, he said, "I've lost some, but not enough" (Brush 2012).
2. The attacks became personal when Senator Rick Jones reacted to Fabiano's post by writing her directly on Facebook, saying "I hear you are taking head meds. Is that true?" (Jones 2011). She filed an ethics complaint against him for cyber bullying, and he subsequently wrote an apology letter (Fabiano 2011a).
3. To determine this number, I searched on Google the name of each person listed in the committee meeting minutes along with the search terms "Michigan" and "tea party."
4. Calculated using the minutes of the following meetings of the House Health Policy Committee: 9/8/2011, 9/15/2011, 10/6/2011, 10/13/2011, 10/20/2011, 10/27/

2011, 11/3/2011, 11/10/2011, 12/1/2011, 1/19/2011, 7/25/2012, and 11/29/2012, all available at House.Michigan.gov. Representative Womack missed 9 of these 12 meetings.

5. Determined using the minutes for each of the meetings for his three committees during this period.

CHAPTER 4

1. According to Gallup State of the States (2010). Idaho is second only to Mississippi in terms of the percentage of residents who describe their political views as conservative. http://www.gallup.com/poll/125066/State-States.aspx. See also Shor and McCarty 2011.
2. Referring to the bills that would be advanced to create an exchange in 2013.
3. A full directory of bills introduced in 2013 is available at http://legislature.idaho.gov/legislation/2013/minidata.htm
4. To verify this point I searched the minutes of every meeting held in 2013 of the nine standing Senate Committees, the 13 standing House Committees, and the Joint Finance and Appropriations Committee. Available at http://legislature.idaho.gov/sessioninfo/2013/standingcommittees/committeeminutes.htm
5. More than one-third of Idaho's legislators in 2013 were Mormon and would likely have recognized this reference. Doctrine and Covenants 8:2 is a prominent verse of Mormon scripture in which Joseph Smith says the Lord explained to him how the Holy Ghost reveals whether something is true. "Behold, I will tell you in your mind and in your heart, by the Holy Ghost, which shall come upon you and which shall dwell in your heart." The subtle implication being that opposing the exchange was God's will.

CHAPTER 5

1. A handful of states explored establishing an exchange while the Supreme Court considered *King v. Burwell*, but no more states followed through as of August 2015.
2. Ultimately such a provision was not required by the federal government, and Democrats would lose ground on this point in 2013.

CHAPTER 6

1. He made this comment as an audience member at event, sponsored by the Scholars Strategy Network, at Harvard University on October 2, 2014.

REFERENCES

American Legislative Exchange Council (ALEC). 2011. "The State Legislator's Guide to Repealing Obamacare." Accessed March 30, 2013. http://www.alec.org/wp-content/uploads/State_Leg_Guide_to_Repealing_ObamaCare.pdf.

Ames, Michael. 2011. "New Poll Has Raul Labrador and Walt Minnick Essentially Tied in Idaho." *Politics Daily*. Accessed April 10, 2014. http://www.politicsdaily.com/2010/10/26/new-poll-has-raul-labrador-and-walt-minnick-tied-in-idaho/.

Apollonio, D and Raymond J. La Raja. 2006. "Term Limits, Campaign Contributions, and the Distribution of Power in State Legislatures." *Legislative Studies Quarterly*. 31(2): 259-281.

Armstrong, Deborah. 2010. "SJM 1 Health Care Reform Working Group." Accessed March 14, 2014. http://www.nmlegis.gov/lcs/fileExists/interimreports/HRWG10.pdf.

Associated Press (AP). 2011a. "Idaho Senate Panel Dumps Health Care Nullification." *Rexburg Standard Journal*, February 25. Accessed April 11, 2014. http://www.rexburgstandardjournal.com/news/idaho-senate-panel-dumps-health-care-nullification/article_f6bb18c8-412b-11e0-9660-001cc4c002e0.html#axzz2qUGJZ8K8.

Associated Press (AP). 2011b. "Michigan Senate Approves Health Exchange Measure." *Bloomberg Businessweek*. Accessed July 12, 2013. http://www.businessweek.com/ap/financialnews/D9QU2HHG0.htm.

Associated Press (AP). 2011c. "Snyder Rep Seeks Way to Get Health Exchange Going." *MLive*. Accessed July 13, 2013. http://www.mlive.com/politics/index.ssf/2011/12/snyder_rep_seeks_way_to_get_he.html.

Associated Press (AP). 2012. "Poll: Many NM Voters Back Medicaid Expansion." *Roswell Daily Record*, September 15. Accessed June 22, 2017. https://rdrnews.com/wordpress/blog/2012/09/15/poll-many-nm-voters-back-medicaid-expansion/

Associated Press (AP). 2013. "AG Jim Hood Says Insurance Commissioner Mike Chaney Can Set Up Health Exchange (updated)." *Gulflive.com*, January 15. Accessed March 2, 2014. http://blog.gulflive.com/mississippi-press-news/2013/01/ag_jim_hood_says_insurance_com.html.

Baerren, Eric. 2012. "Lesia Liss' tremendously awful judgment." *Michiganliberal.com*. Accessed July 12, 2013. http://www.michiganliberal.com/diary/19222/lesia-liss-tremendously-awful-judgment.

Bagley, Nicholas. 2015. "In Ruling on Obamacare Provision, Court Didn't Rewrite Law—It Read It." *Los Angeles Times*, June 25, 2015. Accessed September 30, 2015. http://www.latimes.com/opinion/op-ed/la-oe-0626-bagley-king-burwell-20150626-story.html.

Bagley, Nicholas, and David K. Jones. 2015. "No Good Options: Picking Up the Pieces after King v. Burwell." *Yale Law Journal Forum* 125 (April 29). http://www.

yalelawjournal.org/forum/no-good-options-picking-up-the-pieces-after-king-v-burwell. Accessed September 30, 2015.

Bagley, Nicholas, David K. Jones, and Timothy S. Jost. 2015. "Predicting the Fallout from King v. Burwell—Exchanges and the ACA." *New England Journal of Medicine* 372: 101–104.

Barbour, Haley. 2009. "2009 State of the State Speech." Accessed February 27, 2014. http://www.jacksonfreepress.com/news/2009/jan/13/barbours-2009-state-of-the-state-address/.

Barker, Kim, and Theodoric Meyer. 2014. "The Dark Money Man: How Sean Noble Moved the Kochs' Cash into Politics and Made Millions." *ProPublica*. Accessed April 28, 2014. http://www.propublica.org/article/the-dark-money-man-how-sean-noble-moved-the-kochs-cash-into-politics-and-ma.

Barnett, Jessica C., and Marina S. Vornovitsky. 2016. "Health Insurance Coverage in the United States: 2015." US Census Bureau. Accessed September 28, 2016. http://www.census.gov/content/dam/Census/library/publications/2016/demo/p60-257.pdf.

Barstow, David. 2010. "Tea Party Lights Fuse for Rebellion on Right." *New York Times*, February 15. Accessed April 10, 2014. http://www.nytimes.com/2010/02/16/us/politics/16teaparty.html?pagewanted=all&_r=1&.

Bartels, Larry M. 2006. "What's the Matter with *What's the Matter with Kansas?*" *Quarterly Journal of Political Science* 1: 201–226.

Basham, Patrick. 2011. "Term Limits: A Reform That Works." *Our Generation*. Accessed February 24, 2014. http://ourgeneration.org/wp-content/uploads/2011/06/term-limits.pdf.

Béland, Daniel, Philip Rocco, and Alex Waddan. 2014. "Implementing Health Care Reform in the United States: Intergovernmental Politics and the Dilemmas of Institutional Design." *Health Policy* 116 (1): 51–60.

Béland, Daniel, Philip Rocco, and Alex Waddan. 2016. *Obamacare Wars: Federalism, State Politics, and the Affordable Care Act*. Lawrence: University Press of Kansas.

Berch, Neil. 1992. "Why do some states play the federal-aid game better than others?" *American Politics Quarterly*. Vol. 20(3): 366-377.

Beyle, Thad. 2004. "The Governors," in *Politics in the American States: A Comparative Analysis*. Virginia Gray and Russell L. Hanson eds. 8th Edition. CQ Press: Washington D.C.

Bien, Kristin. 2011. "Rev. Jesse Jackson Speaks to City Leaders in Benton Harbor." *WSBT*. Accessed July 12, 2013. http://articles.wsbt.com/2011-04-20/emergency-financial-manager_29453416.

Bingham, Debra. 2007. "Every Change Needs a Champion." *Journal of Perinatal Education* 16 (3): 8–10.

Bipartisan Government Relations (BGR). 2012. "Governor Haley Barbour Returns to BGR Group." Accessed March 2, 2014. http://www.bgrdc.com/x-news/pressreleases-2012/1-HB-Press-Release.html.

Blake, Aaron. 2010. "Top GOP Recruit Vaughn Ward Loses in Idaho Primary." *The Fix*, May 26. Accessed April 10, 2014. http://voices.washingtonpost.com/thefix/house/top-gop-recruit-vaughn-ward-lo.html.

Blumberg, Linda J., Matthew Buettgens, and John Holahan. 2015. "The Implications of a Supreme Court Finding for the Plaintiff in King v. Burwell: 8.2 Million More Uninsured and 35% Higher Premiums." The Urban Institute. Accessed September 30, 2015. http://www.rwjf.org/content/dam/farm/reports/issue_briefs/2015/rwjf417289.

Blumberg, Linda J., et al. 2014. "Measuring Marketplace Enrollment Relative to Projections." The Urban Institute. http://www.urban.org/sites/default/files/alfresco/publication-pdfs/413087-Measuring-Marketplace-Enrollment-Relative-to-Enrollment-Projections.PDF.

Bolger, Jase. 2012. "Speaker Bolger's Statement on the Future of a Health Exchange in Michigan." Michigan House Republicans. Accessed July 12, 2013. https://www.facebook.com/notes/michigan-house-republicans/news-speaker-bolgers-statement-on-the-future-of-a-health-exchange-in-michigan/10151523769288219.

Bowers, Chris. 2011. "Effort to Recall Michigan Gov. Rick Snyder Comes up Short." *Daily Kos*. Accessed July 12, 2013. http://www.dailykos.com/story/2011/09/28/1021044/-Effort-to-recall-Michigan-Gov-Rick-Snyder-comes-up-short.

Braun, Ken, and Jack McHugh. 2010. "Tea Party Activist Toolbox." Mackinac Center for Public Policy. Accessed July 12, 2013. http://www.mackinac.org/archives/2010/TEApartytoolbox2.pdf.

Brown, Lawrence D. 2010. "Pedestrian Paths: Why Path Dependence Theory Leaves Health Policy Analysis Lost in Space." *Journal of Health Politics, Policy, and Law* 35 (4): 643–661.

Brusk, Steve. 2010. "Pelosi to use historic gavel to preside over vote." *CNN*. Accessed July 6, 2013. http://politicalticker.blogs.cnn.com/2010/03/21/pelosi-to-use-historic-gavel-to-preside-over-reform/.

Bryant, Phil. 2012a. "Governor Bryant Issues Statement on Insurance Exchange." Accessed March 2, 2014. http://www.governorbryant.com/governor-bryant-issues-statement-on-insurance-exchange/.

Bryant, Phil. 2012b. "Letter to Secretary Kathleen Sebelius." Accessed March 2, 2014. http://images.politico.com/global/2012/11/28/bryanthhsletter.html.

Bryant, Phil. 2013a. "Phil Bryant to Secretary Kathleen Sebelius," January 18. Letter. Accessed February 28, 2013. http://www.mid.ms.gov/press_releases/2013/pressrel020813.pdf.

Bryant, Phil. 2013b. "Governor Bryant Issues Statement on Health Care Exchange." Accessed March 2, 2014. http://www.governorbryant.com/governor-bryant-issues-statement-on-health-care-exchange/.

Budoff Brown, Carrie. 2010. "Nelson: National Exchange a Dealbreaker." *Politico*, January 25.

Budoff Brown, Carrie, and Glenn Thrush. 2010. "Nancy Pelosi Steeled White House for Health Push." *Politico*, March 20. Accessed March 20, 2014. http://www.politico.com/news/stories/0310/34753.html.

Bulman-Pozen, Jessica, and Heather K. Gerken. 2009. "Uncooperative Federalism." *Yale Law Journal* 118 (7): 1256–1310.

Burke, Sheila, and Elaine Kamarck, 2013. "Brookings Center for Effective Public Management. The Affordable Care Act: A User's Guide to Implementation." Accessed February 24, 2014. http://www.brookings.edu/~/media/research/files/papers/2013/10/15%20affordable%20care%20act%20user%20guide%20burke%20kamarck/kamarckburkeaca%20user%20guide101513.pdf.

Burns, Gus. 2012. "Metro Cops: State Rep. Jimmy Womack, D-Detroit, Victim of Robbery, Attempted-Carjacking in Detroit." *MLive*. Accessed July 12, 2013. http://detroit.cbslocal.com/2012/07/10/state-lawmaker-robbed-at-gunpoint-near-detroit-home/.

Burns, Nancy, et al. 2008. "Pockets of expertise: Institutional capacity in twentieth-century state legislatures." *Studies in American Political Development*. Vol. 22(2): 229–246.

Callaghan, Timothy, and Lawrence Jacobs. 2016. "Interest Group Conflict over Medicaid Expansion: The Surprising Impact of Public Advocates." *American Journal of Public Health* 106 (2): 308–313.

Camp, Dave. 2013. "Issues: Health." Accessed July 6, 2013. http://camp.house.gov/issues/issue/?IssueID=4630.

Cannon, Michael F. 2011a. "Should Missouri Create a Health Insurance Exchange?" Testimony delivered before the Interim Committee on Health Insurance Exchanges, Missouri Senate, September 15. Accessed March 30, 2013. http://www.cato.org/publications/congressional-testimony/should-missouri-create-health-insurance-exchange.

Cannon, Michael F. 2011b. "Should Virginia Create a Health Insurance Exchange?" Testimony delivered before the Virginia Legislature's Joint Commission on Health Care. June 14. Mackinac Center for Public Policy. Accessed July 12, 2013. http://www.mackinac.org/15237.

Cannon, Michael F. 2013. "50 Vetoes: How States Can Stop the Obama Health Care Law." *Cato Institute*. Accessed April 27, 2014. http://www.cato.org/publications/white-paper/50-vetoes-how-states-can-stop-obama-health-care-law.

Carey, J. M., et al. 2006. "The Effects of Term Limits on State Legislatures: A New Survey of the 50 States." *Legislative Studies Quarterly* 31 (1): 105–134.

Carter, Ted. 2013. "Chaney: Rates to Soar on State Healthcare Exchange." *Mississippi Business Journal*, August 6. Accessed March 2, 2014. http://msbusiness.com/blog/2013/08/06/chaney-rates-to-soar-on-state-healthcare-exchange/.

Cauthon, Phil. 2011a. "A Legislator's Guide to Repealing Obamacare." August 29. Remarks in a video recording of speech recorded by Richard Fry, PatriotCoalition.com. Accessed March 30, 2013. http://www.khi.org/news/2011/aug/29/elements-kansas-policy-mirror-guide-repealing/.

Cauthon, Phil. 2011b. "Are Kansas Officials Studying the ALEC Playbook?" Kansas Health Institute. Accessed February 20, 2013. http://www.khi.org/news/2011/aug/29/elements-kansas-policy-mirror-guide-repealing/.

CBS News. 2010. "Idaho to Sue if Health Care Bill Passes." *CBS News*, March 17. Accessed April 10, 2014. http://www.cbsnews.com/news/idaho-to-sue-if-health-care-bill-passes/.

Center for Budget Policy and Priorities (CBPP). 2013. "Status of State Health Insurance Exchange Implementation." Accessed March 4, 2013. http://www.cbpp.org/files/CBPP-Analysis-on-the-Status-of-State-Exchange-Implementation.pdf.

Centers for Medicare and Medicaid Services (CMS). 2014. "The Center for Consumer Information and Insurance Oversight." Accessed April 10, 2014. http://www.cms.gov/CCIIO/Resources/Marketplace-Grants/id.html.

Centers for Medicare and Medicaid Services (CMS). 2016. "Historical." Accessed June 22, 2017. https://www.cms.gov/research-statistics-data-and-systems/statistics-trends-and-reports/nationalhealthexpenddata/nationalhealthaccountshistorical.html

Chaney, Mike. 2012. "Mississippi Builds Insurance Exchange, Even as it Fights Health Law." *KCUR.org*, March 16, 2012. Accessed March 2, 2014.

Charmaz, Kathy. 2006. *Constructing Grounded Theory*. Thousand Oaks: SAGE Publications.

Cheney, Kyle. 2014. "Mississippi Congressman Sees Racism in Anti-Obamacare Fervor." *Politico*. Accessed May 2, 2014. http://www.politico.com/story/2014/04/report-mississippi-congressman-sees-racism-in-anti-obamacare-fervor-106163.html.

Christoff, Chris. 2010. "State Rep. Jase Bolger to Replace Andy Dillon as House Speaker." Accessed July 6, 2013. http://election2010.illumen.org/latest-news/state-rep-jase-bolger-to-replace-andy-dillon-as-house-speaker.

Citizens United vs. Federal Election Commission. 558 U.S. 310 (2010).

Clouser McCann, Pamela J. 2016. *The Federal Design Dilemma: Congress and Intergovernmental Delegation*. Cambridge: Cambridge University Press.

Coburn, Tom. 2011. "Dr. Coburn Supports State-Based Health Insurance Exchange." Coburn.senate.gov, November 17. Accessed March 30, 2013. http://www.coburn.senate.gov/public/index.cfm/rightnow?ContentRecord_id=b4ccb62e-1ffb-4e77-9325-da0c33e87e67&ContentType_id=b4672ca4-3752-49c3-bffc-fd099b51c966&Group_id=00380921-999d-40f6-a8e3-470468762340.

Cohen, Gary. 2013. "Gary Cohen to Mike Chaney," February 8. Letter. Accessed February 28, 2013. http://www.mid.ms.gov/press_releases/2013/pressrel020813.pdf.

Colbeck, Patrick. 2011. "Colbeck Withdraws Support of Senate Healthcare Exchange Bill." Accessed July 12, 2013. http://www.misenategop.com/senators/readarticle.asp?id=4477&District=7.

Conyers, John. 2013. "Conyers reintroduces national single-payer health care bill." Press release. http://conyers.house.gov/index.cfm/press-releases?ID=6c9a002e-2698-4141-b61a-ec76834c6cc0 Accessed July 6, 2013.

Coughlin, Teresa A. 2012. "ACA Implementation—Monitoring and Tracking New Mexico." *Urban Institute*. Accessed March 14, 2014. http://www.urban.org/UploadedPDF/412642-aca-implementation.pdf.

Cox, Mike. 2010. "Mike Cox 2010 TV Spot 'Mike Cox: Fighter for Life.'" *Mike Cox for Governor*. Accessed July 6, 2013. https://www.youtube.com/watch?v=STbEhdCXakw.

Cutler, David. 2010. "Urgent Need for Changes in Health Reform Implementation." Memo to Larry Summers, May 11. Accessed April 30, 2014. http://www.washingtonpost.com/blogs/wonkblog/files/2013/11/Cutler-implementation-memo-1.pdf.

Cutler, David M., Karen Davis, and Kristof Stremikis. 2010. "The Impact of Health Reform on Health System Spending." *Commonwealth Fund/Center for American Progress*. Accessed April 2, 2013. http://www.commonwealthfund.org/~/media/Files/Publications/Issue%20Brief/2010/May/1405_Cutler_impact_hlt_reform_on_hlt_sys_spending_ib_v4.pdf.

Dao, James. 2006. "Waters Recede, and Popularity Rises." *New York Times*, February 21. Accessed March 2, 2014. http://www.nytimes.com/2006/02/21/world/americas/21iht-barbour.html?_r=2&.

Dingell, John. 2013. "Issues: Health Care." Accessed July 6, 2013. http://dingell.house.gov/issue/health-care.

Donatelli, Frank. 2010. "Number of Party Switchers to GOP in State Legislatures since the Election Now at 25." *LibertarianRepublican.net*, December 29. Accessed March 3, 2013. http://www.libertarianrepublican.net/2010/12/number-of-party-switchers-to-gop-in.html

Donmenech, Ben. 2011. "Barbour Gets It Wrong on Obamacare Exchanges." *Washington Examiner*, February 21. Accessed February 27, 2014. http://washingtonexaminer.com/barbour-gets-it-wrong-on-obamacare-exchanges/article/141164.

Doonan, Michael. 2013. *American Federalism in Practice: The Formulation and Implementation of Contemporary Health Policy*. Washington, D.C.: Brookings Institution Press.

Dooren, Jennifer Corbett. 2013. "Two States Seek Help with Health Exchanges." *Wall Street Journal*. Accessed April 28, 2014. http://online.wsj.com/news/articles/SB10001424127887323336104578499444065609364.

Dukakis, Michael. 2001. "The Governors and health policymaking," in *The New Politics of State Health Policy*. Robert B. Hackey and David A. Rochefort eds. University of Kansas Press: Lawrence.

Eggert, David. 2013. "Michigan Lawmakers Mull $31M for Health Care Exchange." *MLive*. Accessed July 6, 2013. http://www.mlive.com/politics/index.ssf/2013/02/michigan_lawmakers_mull_31m_fo.html.

Ehrenhalt, Alan. 2015. "Why It's Important to Know Your Lawmaker's Day Job." *Governing*. Accessed September 28, 2016. http://www.governing.com/columns/assessments/gov-state-legislator-professions.html.

Epstein, Reid J. 2012. "Republicans Feud over Obamacare." *Politico*, November 2012. Accessed March 2, 2014. http://www.politico.com/story/2012/11/republicans-fight-each-other-over-obamacare-84422.html.

Erler, H. Abbie. 2007. "Legislative Term Limits and State Spending." *Public Choice*. 133(3): 479–494.

Fabiano, Joan. 2011a. "SB 693 Passes—On to the House!" *GrassrootsMichigan.com*. Accessed July 12, 2013. http://grassrootsmichigan.com/?p=1213.

Fabiano, Joan. 2011b. "This Bill Must Be Stopped." *Rightmichigan.com*. Accessed July 12, 2013. http://www.rightmichigan.com/story/2011/12/12/10545/916.

Fabiano, Joan. 2012a. "Final Meeting for Public Testimony on Health Care Exchange (Obama Care)." User: Joan Fabiano. Accessed July 12, 2013. https://www.facebook.com/events/140317816076802/.

Fabiano, Joan. 2012b. "How to Become an Effective Activist—What You Need to Know to Combat the Implementation of a MI Health Care Exchange (Obama Care)." *GrassrootsMichigan.com*. Accessed July 12, 2013. http://grassrootsmichigan.com/?p=1088.

Fabiano, Joan. 2012c. "Michigan ObamaCare UpDate." *GrassrootsMichigan.com*. Accessed July 12, 2013. http://grassrootsmichigan.com/?p=2006.

Fabiano, Joan. 2012d. "Congratulations! Health Care Exchange Bill Defeated, on to Right to Work!" *GrassrootsMichigan.com*. Accessed July 12, 2013. http://grassrootsmichigan.com/?p=2339.

Fox, Daniel M. 2010. *Science and Governance: Research, Health Policy, and American States*. Berkeley: University of California Press.

Gaddis, Mildred. 2010. "Granholm: Health Reform Will Make Michigan Stronger." WCBH News Detroit. Accessed July 6, 2013. http://wchbnewsdetroit.com/264411/granholm-health-reform-will-make-michigan-stronger/.

Gantert, Tom. 2010. "Health Care Freedom Petition Comes up Short." *Michigan Capitol Confidential*. Accessed July 6, 2013. http://www.michigancapitolconfidential.com/13121.

Gautz, Chris. 2012. "Michigan Will Not Have State-Run Health Insurance Exchange." *Crain's Detroit Business*. Accessed July 12, 2013. http://www.crainsdetroit.com/article/20121129/FREE/121129856/michigan-will-not-have-state-run-health-insurance-exchange.

Gavette, William. 2012. "Senate Bill SB 693—Michigan Health Care Exchange." *Lapeer County Tea Party Patriots*. Accessed July 12, 2013. http://lapeerteaparty.ning.com/profiles/blogs/senate-bill-sb-693-michigan-health-care-exchange.

Gem State Tea Party. 2013. "The Gem State Tea Party Confederation." Accessed April 10, 2014. http://www.gstp.org/confederation/.

Gillette, Becky. 2011. "Mississippi ahead of Other States in Developing Health Insurances Exchanges." *Mississippi Medical News*, October 19. Accessed

March 2, 2014. http://mississippimedicalnews.com/mississippi-ahead-of-other-states-in-developing-health-insurance-exchanges-cms-1560.

Gillman, Jason. 2012. "Next Step—Representative Exchange." *Right Michigan*. Accessed July 12, 2013. http://www.rightmichigan.com/story/2012/11/28/232327/29.

Gray, Virginia; David Lowery; and Jennifer K. Benz. 2013. *Interest Groups and Health Care Reform Across the United States*. Georgetown University Press: Washington D.C.

Greenberg, Dan. "Term Limits: The Only Way to Clean Up Congress." The Heritage Foundation, 1994. Accessed February 27, 2014. http://www.heritage.org/research/reports/1994/08/bg994nbsp-term-limitsnbsp-the-only-way.

Greer, Scott L. 2011. "The States' Role Under the Patient Protection and Affordable Care Act." *Journal of Health Politics, Policy and Law* 36: 369–473.

Grogan, Colleen M., and Elizabeth E. Rigby. 2009. "Federalism, Partisan Politics, and Shifting Support for State Flexibility: The Case of the U.S. State Children's Health Insurance Program." *Publius* 39 (1): 47–69.

Hacker, Jacob S. 2008. "The Case for Public Plan Choice in National Health Reform: Key to Cost Control and Quality Coverage." *Institute for America's Future*. Accessed April 2013. http://institute.ourfuture.org/files/Jacob_Hacker_Public_Plan_Choice.pdf.

Hacker, Jacob S. 2009. "Healthy Competition: The Whys and How of Public Plan Choice." *New England Journal of Medicine* 360: 2269–2271.

Haeder, Simon F., and David L. Weimer. 2013. "You Can't Make Me Do It: State Implementation of Insurance Exchanges under the Affordable Care Act." *Public Administration Review*. 73(1):S34–S47.

Haines, Gail. 2010. Legislation sponsored by Representative Gail Haines in the Michigan House of Representatives, 2009–2010. Accessed April 28, 2014. http://www.legislature.mi.gov/(S(v2fp3n55v2om0e55sazq2v45))/mileg.aspx?page=ExecuteSearch&legislativesession=2009-2010&chamber=House&sponsor=Gail%20Haines.

Haislmaier, Edmund. 2006. "The Significance of Massachusetts Health Reform." The Heritage Foundation, April 11. Accessed April 2, 2013. http://www.heritage.org/research/reports/2006/04/the-significance-of-massachusetts-health-reform.

Hamel, Liz, Mira Norton, and Mollyann Brodie. 2015. "Survey of Kentucky Residents on State Health Policy." Kaiser Family Foundation. December 11, 2015. Accessed September 28, 2016. http://kff.org/health-reform/poll-finding/survey-of-kentucky-residents-on-state-health-policy/.

Harkin, Tom. 2013. "Statement by Senator Tom Harkin on the Importance of the Prevention Fund to Save Lives and Money." US Senate Committee on Health, Education, Labor & Pensions. http://www.help.senate.gov/ranking/newsroom/press/statement-by-senator-tom-harkin-on-the-importance-of-the-prevention-fund-to-save-lives-and-money.

Harrison, Bobby. 2012. "Chaney Presses Ahead on Exchange." *DJournal.com*, November 11. Accessed March 2, 2014. http://djournal.com/news/chaney-presses-ahead-on-exchange/.

Hatch, Orrin, Lamar Alexander, and John Barasso. 2015. "We Have a Plan for Fixing Health Care." *The Washington Post*. March 1, 2015. Accessed September 30, 2015. https://www.washingtonpost.com/opinions/we-have-a-plan-for-fixing-health-care/2015/03/01/e0925502-becc-11e4-8668-4e7ba8439ca6_story.html.

Heine, Kevin Rex. 2012. "An Email Sent Out . . ." Comment #7 to a post titled, "Next Step—Representative Exchange," by Jason Gillman. November 28, 2012.

RightMichigan.com. Accessed July 12, 2013. http://www.rightmichigan.com/comments/2012/11/28/232327/29/7#7.

Heinz, John P., et al. 1990. "Inner Circles or Hollow Cores? Elite Networks in National Policy Systems." *Journal of Politics* 52: 356–390.

Hess, Jeffrey. 2011. "Mississippi Tea Party Endorses Phil Bryant." *Mississippi Public Broadcasting (MPB)*. Accessed March 2, 2014. http://mpbonline.org/News/article/mississippi_tea_party_endorses_phil_bryant

Hess, Jeffrey. 2013. "Right-Leaning Think Tank Warns Mississippi Law Makers about State Run Health Insurance Exchange." *Mississippi Public Broadcasting*, January 16. Accessed March 2, 2014. http://mpbonline.org/News/article/right_leaning_think_tank_warns_mississippi_law_markers_about_state_run_heal.

Hill, Austin. 2013. "Senate Approves Otter's State Insurance Exchange on 23-12 Vote." *IdahoReporter.com*. Accessed April 28, 2014. http://www.idahoreporter.com/2013/senate-approves-otters-state-insurance-exchange-on-23-12-vote/.

Hoffman, Kathy Barks. 2012. "Emergency Manager Repeal Effort Takes Step Forward, Board of Canvassers to Vote Tomorrow." *WXYZ.com*. Accessed July 12, 2013. http://www.dailykos.com/story/2012/04/25/1086310/-BREAKING-Enough-signatures-validated-to-put-Mich-Emergency-Manager-law-on-ballot-on-HOLD.

Hood, Jim. 2010. "Hood Says He Won't Be Pressured to Sue over Healthcare Reform." *WILOX 13*, April 7. Accessed February 27, 2014. http://www.wlox.com/Global/story.asp?S=12270422.

Hulse, Carl. 2010. "Idaho 1st District Profile." *New York Times*, December 10. Accessed April 10, 2014. http://elections.nytimes.com/2010/house/idaho/1.

Hurst, Dustin. 2010a. "Otter Signs Idaho Health Freedom Act (video)." *Idaho Reporter.com*, March 17. Accessed April 10, 2014. http://www.idahoreporter.com/2010/otter-signs-idaho-health-freedom-act-video/.

Hurst, Dustin. 2010b. "Pro-Life Group Throws Support behind Labrador." *Idaho Rporter.com*, April 23. Accessed April 10, 2014. http://www.spokesman.com/stories/2013/sep/15/idaho-freedom-foundations-charitable-status/.

Idaho Executive Order No. 2011-03. 2011. Accessed April 11, 2014. http://gov.idaho.gov/pdf/Executive%20Order%202011-03.pdf.

Idaho House Bill 391. 2010. "Idaho Health Freedom Act." Accessed April 10, 2014. http://www.legislature.idaho.gov/legislation/2010/H0391.htm.

Idaho House Bill 179. 2013. "House Bill 179." Accessed April 28, 2014. http://www.legislature.idaho.gov/legislation/2013/H0179.pdf.

Idaho House Health and Welfare Committee. 2013. "Minutes: House Health and Welfare Committee." Accessed April 28, 2014. http://legislature.idaho.gov/sessioninfo/2013/standingcommittees/hhelmin.pdf.

Idaho House of Representatives. 2013. "Journal of the House of Representatives: Organizational Session and First Regular Session of the Sixty-Second Legislature of the State of Idaho." Accessed April 28, 2014. http://legislature.idaho.gov/sessioninfo/2013/Journals/hfinal.pdf.

Idaho Reporter. 2014. "About IFF." *IdahoReporter.com*. Accessed April 28, 2014. http://www.idahoreporter.com/about/.

Idaho Senate Bill 1158. 2011. 61st Legislature. "Appropriations." Available from Idaho State Legislature; Accessed April 10, 2014.

Idaho Senate Bill 1042. 2013. "Idaho Health Insurance Exchange Act." Accessed April 28, 2014. http://legislature.idaho.gov/legislation/2013/S1042.pdf.

Idaho Senate Commerce and Human Resources Committee. 2013. "Minutes: Senate Commerce and Human Resources Committee." Accessed April 28, 2014. http://legislature.idaho.gov/sessioninfo/2013/standingcommittees/scommin.pdf.

Idaho Senate State Affairs Committee. 2010. "January 18 Minutes." Accessed April 10, 2014. http://legislature.idaho.gov/sessioninfo/2010/standingcommittees/sstafmin.pdf.

Idaho Senate State Affairs Committee. 2011. "January 14 Agenda." Accessed April 11, 2014. http://legislature.idaho.gov/sessioninfo/2011/standingcommittees/sstafmin.pdf.

Iler, Eileen. 2012. "Testimony Submitted to the Michigan Committee on Health Policy." January 19. Accessed July 12, 2013. http://www.house.mi.gov/SessionDocs/2011-2012/Testimony/Committee11-1-19-2012.pdf.

Jacobs, Larry R., and Theda Skocpol. 2010. *Health Care Reform and American Politics: What Everyone Needs to Know.* New York: Oxford University Press.

Jacobs, Lawrence, and Timothy Callaghan. 2013. "Why States Expand Medicaid: Party, Resources, and History." *Journal of Health Politics, Policy, and Law* 38 (5): 1023–1050.

Jennings, Trip. 2011. "Lawmakers Still Mulling Health Care Exchange Bill." *Santa Fe New Mexican, March* 2. A-1. Accessed April 28, 2014. http://www.nmlegis.gov/Sessions/11%20Regular/bills/senate/SB0038HVOTE.pdf.

Jennings, Trip. 2012. "Health Care Official Resigns over Perceived Lag in Progress [The Santa Fe New Mexican]." *InsuranceNews.net*, March 24. Accessed March 20, 2014. http://insurancenewsnet.com/oarticle/2012/03/24/health-care-official-resigns-over-perceived-lag-in-progress-%5bthe-santa-fe-new-me-a-336030.html#.UysynPldWEu.

Jones, David K. 2012. "The Fate of Health Reform—What to Expect in 2012." *New England Journal of Medicine* 366: e7.

Jones, David K. 2015. "Obamacare Politics: Lessons from the Kentucky's Governor's Race." *Health Affairs Blog.* http://healthaffairs.org/blog/2015/11/04/obamacare-politics-lessons-from-the-kentucky-governors-race/.

Jones, David K., et al. 2015. "What Are the States Doing to Prepare for King v. Burwell?" *Health Affairs Blog.* June 4, 2015. Accessed September 30, 2015. http://healthaffairs.org/blog/2015/06/04/what-are-the-states-doing-to-prepare-for-king-v-burwell-part-1/.

Jones, David K., Katharine W. V. Bradley, and Jonathan Oberlander. 2014. "Pascal's Wager: Health Insurance Exchanges, Obamacare, and the Republican Dilemma." *Journal of Health Politics, Policy, and Law* 39 (1): 97–137.

Jones, David K., Phillip M. Singer, and John Z. Ayanian. 2014. "The Changing Landscape of Medicaid." *Journal of the American Medical Association.* 311(19):1965–1966.

Jones, David K., and Scott L. Greer. 2013. "State Politics and the Creation of Health Insurance Exchanges." *American Journal of Public Health* 103 (8): e8–e10.

Jones, Rick. 2011. "Facebook Message to Joan Fabiano." Quoted in a letter from Joan Fabiano to Senate Leader Randy Richardville date November 30, 2011. Accessed July 12, 2013. http://www.scribd.com/doc/74856972/Formal-ethics-complaint-against-Senator-Jones.

Jost, Timothy. 2009. "The Public Option and Insurance Exchange in the House Bill." *Health Affairs Blog,* October 30, 2009. Accessed February 20, 2014. http://healthaffairs.org/blog/2009/10/30/the-public-option-and-insurance-exchange-in-the-house-bill/.

Jost, Timothy S. 2010. "Implementation and Enforcement of Health Care Reform—Federal versus State Government." *New England Journal of Medicine* 362: e2.

Jost, Timothy S. 2013. "Implementing Health Reform: Navigator Grants." *Health Affairs Blog*, August 16, 2013. Accessed September 30, 2015. http://healthaffairs.org/blog/2013/08/16/implementing-health-reform-navigator-grants/.

Jost, T. S., et al. 2015. *Brief of Health Care Policy History Scholars as Amici Curiae Supporting Respondents*. Supreme Court of the United States, No. 14-114.

Kaiser Family Foundation (KFF). 2010. "Kaiser Health Tracking Poll: June 2010." Accessed April 2, 2013. http://www.kff.org/kaiserpolls/upload/8082-C.pdf.

Kaiser Family Foundation (KFF). 2014a. "Total Exchange Grants." Accessed April 27, 2014. http://kff.org/health-reform/state-indicator/total-exchange-grants/. Accessed April 27, 2014.

Kaiser Family Foundation (KFF). 2014b. "State Decisions for Creating Health Insurance Exchanges." Accessed April 25, 2014. http://kff.org/health-reform/state-indicator/health-insurance-exchanges/.

Kaiser Family Foundation (KFF). 2014c. "Marketplace Enrollment as a Share of the Potential Marketplace Population." Accessed May 2, 2014. http://kff.org/health-reform/state-indicator/marketplace-enrollment-as-a-share-of-the-potential-marketplace-population/.

Kaplan, Thomas. 2012. "Cuomo Acts to Advance Health Law in New York." *New York Times*, April 12. Accessed April 2, 2013. http://www.nytimes.com/2012/04/13/nyregion/cuomo-orders-health-insurance-exchange-in-new-york.html.

Keiser, Lael R., and Joe Soss. 1998. "With Good Cause: Bureaucratic Discretion and the Politics of Child Support Enforcement." *American Journal of Political Science* 42 (4): 1133–1156.

Keyes, Scott. 2010. "Cox Becomes Third Health Care Plaintiff to Lose Gubernatorial Bid." *ThinkProgress.org*. Accessed July 6, 2013. http://thinkprogress.org/politics/2010/08/04/111453/cox-health-care-sue/?mobile=nc.

King v. Burwell, 576. U.S. (2015).

Klein, Ezra. 2015. "Republicans Say They Have a Plan if the Supreme Court Rules Against Obamacare. They Don't." *Vox*. Accessed September 30, 2015. http://www.vox.com/2015/3/1/8131269/republicans-obamacare-supreme-court.

Kliff, Sarah. 2011. "Oklahoma Governor Returns $54M Health Care Grant." *Politico*, April 14. Accessed April 2, 2013. http://www.politico.com/news/stories/0411/53216.html.

Koller, Christopher F. "They Called It Secret, We Call It Confidential." *Millbank Memorial Fund: View from Here*. September 2015. Accessed September 30, 2015. http://www.milbank.org/the-view-from-here/they-called-it-secret-we-call-it-confidential.

Kopan, Tal. 2013. "Report: Think Tanks Tied to Kochs." *Politico*. Accessed April 28, 2014. http://www.politico.com/story/2013/11/koch-brothers-think-tank-report-99791.html.

Kousser, Thad. 2004. *Term Limits and the Dismantling of State Legislative Professionalism*. Cambridge: Press Syndicate of the University of Cambridge.

Kousser, Thad, and Justin H. Phillips. 2012. *The Power of American Governors: Winning on Budgets and Losing on Policy*. Cambridge, UK: Cambridge University Press.

Kremer, Amy Saylors. 2009. "Nationwide Chicago Tea Party." Lansing Michigan Tea Party Facebook page. Accessed July 6, 2013. https://www.facebook.com/events/51009926733/.

Lazarus, Jeffrey. 2006. "Term Limits' Multiple Effects on State Legislators' Career Decisions." *State Politics and Policy Quarterly* 6: 357–383.

Luke, Peter. 2011. "Gov. Rick Snyder Signs Michigan Business/Income Tax Overhaul into Law." *MLive*. Accessed July 12, 2013. http://www.mlive.com/politics/index.ssf/2011/05/gov_rick_snyder_signs_michigan.html.

Maddow, Rachel. 2011. "Maddow on Emergency Takeover of Benton Harbor, MI." User: WeAreThePeopleMich. Accessed July 12, 2013. https://www.youtube.com/watch?v=oBzkuiD6LD0

Manna, Paul. 2010. *Collision Course: Federal Education Policy Meets State and Local Realities*. Washington DC: CQ Press.

Martinez, Susana. 2011. "Senate Executive Message No. 53," April 8. Letter. Accessed March 20, 2013. http://www.governor.state.nm.us/uploads/FileLinks/1ea65343013a47f9a948cb019fc237b5/SenateExecutiveMessage53.pdf.

Martinez, Susana. 2014a. "Governor Susana Martinez Delivers State of the State Address." Accessed April 28, 2014. http://governor.state.nm.us/uploads/PressRelease/191a415014634aa89604e0b4790e4768/Governor_Susana_Martinez_Delivers_State_of_the_State_Address.pdf

Martinez, Susana. 2014b. "Cooperative Agreement to Support Establishment of State Operated Health Insurance Exchanges." Accessed June 22, 2017. http://www.scribd.com/doc/254484445/New-Mexico-Health-Exchange-Application-November-2014.

Masket, Seth E., and Jeffrey B. Lewis. 2007. "A Return to Normalcy? Revisiting the Effects of Term Limits on Competitiveness and Spending in California Assembly Elections." *State Politics and Policy Quarterly* 7 (1): 20–38.

McClean, Jim. 2010. "Praeger Gets Green Light to Proceed with Reform." *Kansas Health Institute*. Accessed October 28, 2014. http://www.khi.org/news/2010/dec/09/praeger-given-green-light-proceed-reform-implement/.

McDonough, J. E. 2011. *Inside National Health Reform*. Berkeley: University of California Press.

McDonough, J. E., and McGrath, R. 2001. "State Legislatures and Health Policy in the Market Era." In *The New Politics of State Health Policy*, edited by Robert H. Hackey and David A. Rochefort. Lawrence: University of Kansas Press.

McDonough, John E., Brian Rosman, Fawn Phelps, and Melissa Shannon. 2006. "The Third Wave of Massachusetts Health Care Reform." *Health Affairs* 26: w420–431.

McGillivary, Brian. 2012. "Schmidt and Gillman Square Off in Primary." *Traverse City Record Eagle*. Accessed July 12, 2013. http://record-eagle.com/local/x1447685519/Schmidt-and-Gillman-square-off-in-primary/stripped?device=mobile.

McGrath, Robert J. 2009. "Implementation Theory Revisited . . . Again: Lessons from the State Children's Health Insurance Program." *Politics and Policy* 37(2): 309–336.

McGuinn, Patrick J. 2006. *No Child Left Behind and the Transformation of Federal Education Policy, 1965–2005*. Lawrence: University Press of Kansas.

McHugh, Jack. 2011a. "Creating Health 'Exchange' Entrenches Obamacare." *Mackinac Center for Public Policy*. Accessed July 12, 2013. http://www.mackinac.org/15767.

McHugh, Jack. 2011b. "Gov. Snyder's 'Exchange' an Obamacare Trojan Horse?" Mackinac Center for Public Policy. Accessed July 12, 2013. http://www.mackinac.org/15764.

McHugh, Jack. 2011c. "Michigan Creeps Closer to Obamacare 'Exchange.'" Mackinac Center for Public Policy. Accessed July 12, 2013. http://www.mackinac.org/15501.

McHugh, Jack. 2011d. "Commentary: Obamacare Arrives." *Michigan Capitol Confidential*. Accessed July 12, 2013. http://www.michigancapitolconfidential.com/16102.

Medoff, Marshall H, Christopher Dennis, and Kerri Stephens. 2011. "The Impact of Party Control on the Diffusion of Parental Involvement Laws in the U.S. States." *State Politics and Policy Quarterly* 11 (3): 325–347.

Michigan Chamber of Commerce. 2011. "Michigan Chamber responds to Gov. Snyder's Special Message on Health Care." Accessed July 12, 2013. http://www.michamber.com/news/michigan-chamber-responds-gov-snyders-special-message-health-care.

Michigan Department of State. 2013. "Elections in Michigan: Previous Election Information." Michigan Secretary of State. Accessed July 6, 2013. http://www.mi.gov/sos/0,4670,7-127-1633_8722---,00.html.

Michigan Executive Order No. 2010-4. Accessed October 29, 2014. http://www.legislature.mi.gov/documents/2009-2010/executiveorder/htm/2010-EO-04.htm.

Michigan House Health Policy Committee (MI HHEAL). 2011a. "Minutes of the House Standing Committee on Health Policy." 96th Legislature, 1st Regular Session, September 8, 2011. Accessed July 12, 2013. http://www.house.michigan.gov/SessionDocs/2011-2012/Minutes/HEAL090811.pdf.

Michigan House Health Policy Committee (HHEAL). 2011b. "Minutes of the House Standing Committee on Health Policy." 96th Legislature, 1st Regular Session, September 15, 2011. Accessed July 12, 2013. http://www.house.michigan.gov/SessionDocs/2011-2012/Minutes/HEAL091511.pdf.

Michigan House Health Policy Committee (HHEAL). 2011c. "Minutes of the House Standing Committee on Health Policy." 96th Legislature, 1st Regular Session, October 20, 2011. Accessed July 12, 2013. http://house.michigan.gov/SessionDocs/2011-2012/Minutes/HEAL102011.pdf.

Michigan House Health Policy Committee (HHEAL). 2011d. "Minutes of the House Standing Committee on Health Policy." 96th Legislature, 1st Regular Session, December 1, 2011. http://house.michigan.gov/SessionDocs/2011-2012/Minutes/HEAL120111.pdf Accessed July 12, 2013.

Michigan House Health Policy Committee (HHEAL). 2012a. "Minutes of the House Standing Committee on Health Policy." 96th Legislature, 2nd Regular Session, July 25. Accessed July 12, 2013. http://house.michigan.gov/SessionDocs/2011-2012/Minutes/HEAL072512.pdf.

Michigan House Health Policy Committee (HHEAL). 2012b. "Minutes of the House Standing Committee on Health Policy." 96th Legislature, 2nd Regular Session, November 29. Accessed October 29, 2014. http://house.michigan.gov/SessionDocs/2011-2012/Minutes/HEAL112912.pdf.

Michigan House Bill (HB) 4111 (As Passed House; Version Date: 2/28/13). Michigan Legislature. Accessed March 13, 2013.

Michigan House Roll Call #422. 2011. House Bill 5014, entitled. Accessed July 12, 2013. http://www.legislature.mi.gov/(S(j3il0i453ugchontfqfvst45))/documents/2011-2012/Journal/House/pdf/2011-HJ-10-19-083.pdf.

Michigan House Roll Call #570. 2011. House Bill 5014, entitled. Accessed July 12, 2013. http://www.legislature.mi.gov/(S(ooetq445gufc22uyydasjo45))/documents/2011-2012/Journal/House/pdf/2011-HJ-12-13-100.pdf.

Michigan Legislative Directory. 2011. "Former State Legislatures, 1835–2010." Accessed July 6, 2013. http://www.legislature.mi.gov/(S(tsro2afe1gdyxm3hx5tffszg))/documents/2011-2012/michiganmanual/2011-MM-P0315-p0319.pdf.

Michigan Senate Health Policy Committee (SHEAL). 2011. "Minutes of the Joint Meeting of the Senate Committees on Health Policy and Insurance." 96th

Legislature, 1st Regular Session, July 13, 2011. Accessed July 12, 2013. http://senate.michigan.gov/committees/files/2011-scm-hp__-07-13-1.pdf

Michigan Senate Resolution 95 (SR-95). 2011. As adopted by the Senate, November 10, 2011. Accessed July 12, 2013. http://www.legislature.mi.gov/documents/2011-2012/resolutionadopted/senate/htm/2011-SAR-0095.htm.

Michigan Senate Roll Call #663. 2011. SB 693. Accessed July 12, 2013. http://www.legislature.mi.gov/(S(s3gusvaliq1tmf45i0udgan1))/documents/2011-2012/Journal/Senate/pdf/2011-SJ-11-10-091.pdf.

Michigan Senate Roll Call #664. 2011. SB 693. Accessed July 12, 2013. http://www.legislature.mi.gov/(S(s3gusvaliq1tmf45i0udgan1))/documents/2011-2012/Journal/Senate/pdf/2011-SJ-11-10-091.pdf.

Michigan Senate Roll Call # 675. 2011. HB 5014. Accessed July 12, 2013. http://www.legislature.mi.gov/(S(s3gusvaliq1tmf45i0udgan1))/documents/2011-2012/Journal/Senate/pdf/2011-SJ-11-10-091.pdf.

Michigan Senate Roll Call #792. 2011. HB 5014. Accessed July 12, 2013. http://www.legislature.mi.gov/(S(ooetq445gufc22uyydasjo45))/documents/2011-2012/Journal/Senate/pdf/2011-SJ-12-14-099.pdf.

Michiganvotes.com. 2012. "Michigan Tea Party scorecard—Release 3—Jan 2011 through March 2012." Mackinac Center for Public Policy. Accessed July 13, 2013. http://www.michiganvotes.org/VotingIndex.aspx?ID=736

Miga, Andrew, and Steve LeBlanc. 2012. "Romney's CEO Style Rankled Mass Lawmakers." *U.S. News and World Report*. August 8, 2012. Accessed September 28, 2016. http://www.usnews.com/news/politics/articles/2012/08/02/romneys-ceo-style-rankled-mass-lawmakers.

Millman, Jason. 2013. "Mississippi Insurance Commissioner's Affordable Care Act Plan." *Politico*, July 29. Accessed March 2, 2014. http://www.politico.com/story/2013/07/obamacare-mississippi-health-care-exchange-94842.html.

Mississippi Center for Public Policy (MCPP). 2012. "Mississippi Fast-Tracking 'ObamaCare' Exchange for 2012." Accessed March 2, 2014. http://www.mspolicy.org/mcpp_reports/mcpp_reports_view.php?entryID=319.

Mississippi House Bill 1220. 2011. "Mississippi Health Insurance Benefit Exchange Act; Create" (As Introduced). Mississippi Legislature. Accessed February 27, 2014.

Mississippi Insurance Department (MID). 2012a. "Mississippi Insurance Department Bulletin 2011-9." Accessed March 2, 2014. http://www.mid.ms.gov/bulletins/20119bul.pdf

Mississippi Insurance Department (MID). 2012b. "Mississippi Health Insurance Exchange Advisory Board Meeting." Accessed March 2, 2014. https://www.mid.ms.gov/pdf/ExcAdvBoardMtgMinutes07112012.pdf

Mississippi Insurance Department (MID). 2012c. "Exchange Declaration Letter for the State of Mississippi." Accessed March 2, 2014. http://www.mid.ms.gov/pdf/ExchDecLtr.pdf

Mississippi Insurance Department (MID). 2013. "Official Statement from Mississippi Insurance Commissioner Mike Chaney." Accessed March 2, 2014. http://www.mid.ms.gov/press_releases/2013/pressrel020813.pdf

Mississippi PEP. 2013. "Central Mississippi TEA Party Releases Statement on Rejection of State-Run Health Care Exchange." *Mississippi Pep*, February 8. Accessed March 2, 2014. http://mississippipep.wordpress.com/2013/02/08/central-mississippi-tea-party-releases-statement-on-rejection-of-state-run-health-care-exchange/.

MississippiPolicy. 2012a. "Michael Cannon—States Can Resist Obamacare" (1 of 7). Retrieved from http://www.youtube.com/watch?v=y1EenfaE79U.

MississippiPolicy. 2012b. "Cannon and Chaney Debate ObamaCare and Insurance Exchanges." Retrieved from http://www.youtube.com/watch?v=zE5c0WiuwRA.

MississippiPolicy. 2013. "Chaney Press Conference on Obamacare Exchange." Retrieved from http://www.youtube.com/watch?v=5Be85rPTD5E.

Mississippi Secretary of State. 2008. "2008 Election Results." Accessed April 28, 2014. http://www.sos.state.ms.us/elections/2008/08%20Certification%20Results/Cert/President%20&%20VP.pdf.

Mississippi Secretary of State. 2011. "Official Tabulation of Vote for State Office of Commissioner of Insurance." Accessed March 2, 2014. http://www.sos.ms.gov/links/elections/results/statewide/Insurance%20Commissioner_Statewide%20-%20General%20Election%202011%20Results.pdf.

Mississippi Secretary of State. 2012. "2012 Election Results." Accessed April 28, 2014. http://www.sos.ms.gov/elections/electionresults/2012General/certified%20results/President%20and%20Vice%20President.pdf.

Mississippi Senate Bill 2464. 2014. "Health Insurance Exchange; prohibit State of Mississippi from Establishing." (As Introduced). Mississippi Legislature. Accessed February 27, 2014. http://billstatus.ls.state.ms.us/documents/2014/html/SB/2400-2499/SB2464IN.htm.

Mississippi Senate Bill 2668. 2009. "MS Health Insurance Exchange Act, enact." (As Passed in the Senate). Mississippi Legislature. Accessed February 27, 2014. http://billstatus.ls.state.ms.us/documents/2009/html/SB/2600-2699/SB2668CS.htm.

Mississippi Senate Bill 2833. 2008. "Mississippi Health Insurance Exchange Act of 2008." Mississippi Legislature. Accessed February 27, 2014. http://billstatus.ls.state.ms.us/documents/2008/html/SB/2800-2899/SB2833IN.htm.

Mississippi Senate Bill 2842. 2009. "Comprehensive Health Insurance Risk Pool Association; Revise Provisions of Law Regarding." (Current). Mississippi State Legislature. Accessed March 2, 2014. http://billstatus.ls.state.ms.us/documents/2009/html/SB/2800-2899/SB2842PS.htm.

Mississippi Senate Bill 2992. 2011. "Mississippi Health Benefit Exchange Act; create." (As Introduced). Mississippi Legislature. Accessed February 27, 2014. http://billstatus.ls.state.ms.us/documents/2011/html/SB/2900-2999/SB2992PS.htm.

Mississippi State Personnel Board. 2012. "Personal Services Contract Review Board Rules and Regulations." Accessed March 2, 2014. http://www.mspb.ms.gov/media/2850/pscrb%20rules%20and%20regs%20february%202012.pdf.

Mississippi State Personnel Board. 2013. "Personal Service Contract Review Board." Accessed March 2, 2014. http://www.mspb.ms.gov/personal-service-contract-review-board.aspx.

Mooney, Christopher Z. 2005. "The Impact of State Legislative Term Limits on Lobbyists and Interest Groups." Presented at the 5th Annual State Politics and Policy Conference, May 2005. Accessed April 28, 2014. http://www.polisci.msu.edu/sppc2005/papers/friam/Mooney%20SPPC%202005.pdf.

Mooney, Christopher Z. 2009. "Term Limits as a Boon to Legislative Scholarship: A Review." *State Politics and Policy Quarterly* 9 (2): 204–228.

Mooney, Kevin. 2011. "ObamaCare Opponents Differ Sharply over Strategy at ALEC Conference." *The Pelican Post*, August 8. Accessed April 2, 2013.

http://www.thepelicanpost.org/2011/08/08/obamacare-opponents-differ-sharply-over-strategy-at-alec-conference.

Mudgett, Kate. 2011. "Thousands Protest Gov. Snyder's Budget and Emergency Financial Manager Act at Capitol." *Lansing Star*. Accessed July 12, 2013. http://www.cm-life.com/2011/03/18/protests-a-sign-the-governor-legislature-overstepped-democratic-boundaries-with-new-law/.

Murdock, Richard. 2012. "MAHP Agrees with Gov. Snyder: Exchange Bill Needed Now to Ensure Proper IT Operation." *Michigan Association of Health Plans*. Press release. Accessed July 13, 2013. http://www.mahp.org/media/articles/MAHP%20supports%20Gov.%20Snyder%20on%20exchange.pdf.

Murphy, Brian. 2011. "Senate Passes Department of Insurance Budget with 2.5 Million in Federal Money for Health Exchange." *Idaho Statesman*, March 16, 2011. Accessed April 11, 2014. http://voices.idahostatesman.com/2011/03/16/idahopolitics/senate_passes_department_insurance_budget_with_25_million_federa.

Myers, Laura. 2012. "Republican Governors Meet in Las Vegas." *Review Journal*, November 14. Accessed March 2, 2014. http://www.reviewjournal.com/news/government/republican-governors-meet-las-vegas.

Nather, D. 2012. "John Boehner: 'Obamacare Is the Law of the Land.'" *Politico*. November 8, 2012. Accessed December 15, 2012. http://www.politico.com/news/stories/1112/83605.html.

National Council of State Legislatures (NCSL). 2009. "Size of Legislative Staff." http://www.ncsl.org/research/about-state-legislatures/staff-change-chart-1979-1988-1996-2003-2009.aspx#Session.

National Conference of State Legislatures (NCSL). 2010a. "2010 Post-Election Party Control of State Legislatures." Accessed March 14, 2014. http://www.ncsl.org/research/elections-and-campaigns/2010-postelection-control-of-legislatures.aspx?stateid=nm#data.

National Conference of State Legislatures (NCSL). 2011. *Affordable Care Act: State Action Newsletter*. Accessed April 2, 2013. www.ncsl.org/issues-research/health/affordable-care-act-state-action-newsletter-6.aspx.

National Conference of State Legislatures (NCSL). 2013. "The Term Limited States." Accessed February 20, 2014. http://www.ncsl.org/research/about-state-legislatures/chart-of-term-limits-states.aspx.

National Federal of Independent Businesses (NFIB). 2012. "Small Businesses Divided on Health Care Exchange." Accessed July 13, 2013. http://www.nfib.com/nfib-in-my-state/nfib-in-my-state-content?cmsid=61495.

National Federation of Independent Businesses (NFIB) et al. v. Kathleen Sebelius. 567 U.S. (2012).

National Governors Association (NGA). 2011. "2011 Gubernatorial Election Information." Accessed February 27, 2014. http://www.nga.org/cms/home/governors/elections/col2-content/past-election-information/2011-gubernatorial-election.html.

National Institute on Money in State Politics (NIMSP). 2012. "Idaho Election Overview." Accessed October 30, 2014. http://www.followthemoney.org/election-overview?s=ID&y=2012.

New Mexico Department of Human Services. 2012. "New Mexico Level I Health Insurance Exchange Establishment Grant." Accessed March 20, 2014. https://www.statereforum.org/sites/default/files/nm_health_insurance_exchange_establishment_grant.pdf.

New Mexico Executive Order 2010-032. 2010. "Establishing the New Mexico Office of Health Care Reform and Expanding the Health Care Reform Leadership Team to Facilitate Implementation of Federal Health Care Reform." Accessed March 14, 2014.http://www.democracyfornewmexico.com/files/executiveorderhcr.pdf.
New Mexico Health Care Reform Leadership Team 2010. "Implementing Federal Health Care Reform—A Roadmap for New Mexico." Accessed March 14, 2014. http://www.statecoverage.org/files/NM_-__Federal_Health_Care_Reform_Strategic_Plan_June_2010.pdf.
New Mexico House Bill 1045. 2007. "Health Insurance Exchange Act." Accessed April 28, 2014. http://www.nmlegis.gov/lcs/legislation.aspx?Chamber=H&LegType=B&LegNo=1045&year=07.
New Mexico House Bill 33. 2011. "New Mexico Health Insurance Exchange Act." (Introduced; Version Date: 12/23/10). New Mexico State Legislature. Accessed March 14, 2014.
New Mexico House Health, Government & Indian Affairs Committee. 2013a. "House Bill 168." Accessed April 28, 2014. http://www.nmlegis.gov/Sessions/13%20Regular/bills/house/HB0168GU1.html.
New Mexico House Health, Government & Indian Affairs Committee. 2013b. "Senate Corporations and Transportation Committee Substitute for Senate Public Affairs Committee Substitute for Senate Bill 221 & Senate Public Affairs Committee Substitute for Senate Bill 589." Accessed April 28, 2014. http://www.nmlegis.gov/Sessions/13%20Regular/bills/senate/SB0221GU1.html.
New Mexico House Judiciary Committee. 2013. "House Bill 168." Accessed April 28, 2014. http://www.nmlegis.gov/Sessions/13%20Regular/bills/house/HB0168JC1.html.
New Mexico House of Representatives Roll Call #3293. 2011. "Final Vote Results for SB 38 and 370." Accessed March 20, 2014. http://www.nmlegis.gov/Sessions/11%20Regular/bills/senate/SB0038HVOTE.pdf.
New Mexico House of Representatives Roll Call #3928. 2013. "Final Vote Results for HB 168/A." Accessed March 20, 2014. http://www.nmlegis.gov/Sessions/13%20regular/votes/HB0168HVOTE.pdf.
New Mexico Legislative Health and Human Services Interim Committee. 2012. "Interim Report." Accessed April 28, 2014. http://www.nmlegis.gov/lcs/fileExists/interimreports/LHHS12.pdf.
New Mexico Office of Health Reform. 2010. "New Mexico's Office of Health Care Reform Transition Plan." Accessed March 14, 2014. https://www.statereforum.org/system/files/ohcr_transition_plan_122710.pdf.
New Mexico Secretary of State. 2012. "2012 Official General Election Results." Accessed April 28, 2014. http://www.sos.state.nm.us/uploads/files/Pages%20from%20ALLNMG12%20CAN%20STATEWIDE.pdf.
New Mexico Senate Bill 976. 2007. "Health Insurance Exchange Act." Accessed April 28, 2014. http://www.nmlegis.gov/lcs/legislation.aspx?Chamber=S&LegType=B&LegNo=976&year=07.
New Mexico Senate Bill 38. 2011. "New Mexico Health Insurance Exchange Act." (Introduced; Version Date: 2/23/10). New Mexico State Legislature. Accessed March 14, 2014. https://legiscan.com/NM/bill/SB38/2011.
New Mexico Senate Bill 370. 2011. "New Mexico Health Exchange Act." (Introduced; Version Date: 2/01/11). New Mexico State Legislature. Accessed March 14, 2014. https://legiscan.com/NM/drafts/SB370/2011.

New Mexico Senate Bill 221. 2013. "New Mexico Health Insurance Exchange Act." (First Amendment; Version Date: 3/11/13). New Mexico Legislature. Accessed March 20, 2014. https://legiscan.com/NM/drafts/SB221/2013.

New Mexico Senate Corporations and Transportation Committee. 2013. "Official Roll Call: Substitute for Senate Public Affairs Committee Substitute for Senate Bill 221 and Senate Public Affairs Committee Substitute for Senate Bill 589, as amended, with Emergency Clause." Accessed March 20, 2014. http://www.nmlegis.gov/Sessions/13%20regular/votes/SB0221SVOTE.pdf.

New Mexico Senate Roll Call #215. 2011. "Senate Corporations and Transportation Committee Substitute for Senate Bills 38 & 370, as Amended, with Emergency Clause." Accessed March 14, 2014. http://www.nmlegis.gov/Sessions/11%20Regular/bills/senate/SB0038SVOTE.pdf.

New Mexico Senate Roll Call #4237. 2013a. "SCTCS ETC & SB 221 &589/A/EC." Accessed March 20, 2014. http://www.nmlegis.gov/Sessions/13%20regular/votes/SB0221HVOTE.pdf.

News on 6. 2010. "Idaho Enacts Health Care Freedom Act." *NewsOn6*, March 18. Accessed April 10, 2014. http://www.newson6.com/story/12163750/idaho-enacts-health-care-freedom-act?clienttype=printable.

Nicholson, Roy. 2013. "Chairman's Report." Accessed April 28, 2014. http://msteaparty.ning.com/?xg_source=msg_mes_network.

Nicholson-Crotty, Sean. 2012. "Leaving Money on the Table: Learning from Recent Refusals of Federal Grants in the American States." *Oxford Journals* 42 (3): 449–466.

Oberlander, Jonathan. 2003. *The Political Life of Medicare*. Chicago: University of Chicago Press.

Oberlander, Jonathan, and David K. Jones. 2015. "The Children's Cliff—Extending CHIP." *New England Journal of Medicine* 372: 1979–1981.

Olson, Sean. 2011. "Governor Signs Letter on Health Reform." University of New Mexico, June 17, 2011. Accessed March 20, 2014. https://www.unm.edu/news/2011/june/17gov.html.

Olszewski, Janet. 2010. "The Patient Protection and Affordable Care Act: Michigan's Strategic Plan." Health Insurance Reform Coordinating Council. Accessed july 6, 2013. http://www.michigan.gov/documents/healthcarereform/MIchigan_Strategic Plan 340371_7.pdf.

Ortiz y Pino, Jerry. 1993. "Why New Mexicare Died . . . And Why I Care." *Santa Fe Reporter*, February 24. Accessed March 14, 2014. http://www.newspapers.com/newspage/7692062/.

Otter, C. L. Butch. 2010. "Governor C.L. 'Butch' Otter 2010 State of the State and Budget Address." Accessed April 10, 2014. http://gov.idaho.gov/mediacenter/speeches/sp_2010/FY2010StateofStateSpeech.pdf.

Otter, C. L. Butch. 2011a. "Governor C.L. 'Butch' Otter 2011 State of the State and Budget Address." Accessed April 10, 2014. http://www.gov.idaho.gov/mediacenter/speeches/sp_2011/State_of_the_State_2011.pdf.

Otter, C. L. Butch. 2011b. "C.L. Otter to Honorable Ben Ysursa." April 20. Letter. Accessed April 11, 2014. http://gov.idaho.gov/pdf/House%20Bill%20298%20Veto%20Letter%202011.pdf.

Otter, C. L. Butch. 2011c. "News Release: Governor's Executive Order Prohibits State Agencies from Implementing Obamacare." Accessed April 11, 2014. http://gov.idaho.gov/mediacenter/press/pr2011/prapr11/pr_028.html.

Otter, C. L. Butch. 2013. "State of the State and Budget Address." January 7, 2013. Accessed February 28, 2013. http://gov.idaho.gov/mediacenter/speeches/sp_2013/State%20of%20the%20State%202013.pdf.

Patashnik, E. 2008. *Reforms at Risk: What Happens after Major Policy Changes Are Enacted.* Princeton, NJ: Princeton University Press.

Pear, Robert. 2012. "Romney Aide Helps States Comply with Health Care Law." *New York Times*, July 21. Accessed March 2, 2014. http://www.nytimes.com/2012/07/22/us/politics/romney-aide-leavitt-advises-states-to-prepare-health-care-plans.html?_r=1&.

Pear, Robert. 2013. "States Will Be Given Extra Time to Set Up Health Insurance Exchanges." *New York Times*, January 14. Accessed February 28, 2013. http://www.nytimes.com/2013/01/15/us/states-will-be-given-extra-time-to-set-up-health-insurance-exchanges.html?emc=tnt&tntemail0=y&_r=2&wpisrc=nl_wonk&.

Pender, Geoff. 2012. "Mississippi Tea Party Vows to Fight 'Chaney/Obamacare' Health Insurance Exchange." *Clarionledger.com*, December 4. Accessed March 2, 2014. http://www.clarionledger.com/article/20121204/NEWS/121204009?cid=dlvr.it&gcheck=1&nclick_check=1.

Peterson, Karen. 1994. "Critics Argue Health Plan Isn't Enough." *Santa Fe New Mexican*, February 20, B1. Accessed April 28, 2014. http://search.proquest.com/docview/331393700.

Pettus, Emily Wagster. 2013a. "Mike Chaney Letter to Gov. Phil Bryant Intensifies Mississippi Health Insurance Dispute." *Gulflive.com*, January 4. Accessed March 2, 2014. http://blog.gulflive.com/mississippi-press-news/2013/01/mike_chaney_letter_to_gov_phil.html.

Pettus, Emily Wagster. 2013b. "APNewsBreak: Mississippi Gets OK for Business Exchange." *Bloomberg Businessweek*, October 2. Accessed March 2, 2014. http://www.businessweek.com/ap/2013-10-02/apnewsbreak-miss-dot-gets-ok-for-business-exchange.

Pilkington, Ed. 2016. "Because Scott Walker Asked." *The Guardian*. https://www.theguardian.com/us-news/ng-interactive/2016/sep/14/john-doe-files-scott-walker-corporate-cash-american-politics?CMP=Share_iOSApp_Other.

Plunkett, B. Keith. 2012. "Haley Barbour's Previous Position(s) on Mississippi's Health Insurance Exchange No Longer a Factor. This Is Chaney's Baby Now." *Mississippi Pep*, July 25, 2012. Accessed March 2, 2014. http://mississippipep.wordpress.com/2012/07/25/haley-barbours-positions-on-mississippis-health-insurance-exchange-why-should-we-give-a-damn/.

Popkey, Dan. 2013. "New Health Exchange Bill up for Introduction Wednesday in Idaho House." *The Idaho Statesman*, February 12. Accessed April 28, 2014. http://blogs.idahostatesman.com/new-health-exchange-bill-up-for-introduction-wednesday-in-idaho-house/.

Posner, Paul. 2007. "The Politics of Coercive Federalism in the Bush Era." *Publius—The Journal of Federalism* 37 (3): 390–412.

Powell, Richard J. 2000. "The Impact of Term Limits on the Candidacy Decisions of State Legislators in US House Elections." *Legislative Studies Quarterly*. 25(4):645–661.

Pradhan, Rachana. 2015. "A State Fix if Court Hits Obamacare?" *Politico*. June 17, 2015. Accessed September 30, 2015. http://www.politico.com/story/2015/06/a-state-fix-if-court-hits-obamacare-119089.

Pressman, Jeffrey L., and Aaron Wildavsky. 1979. *Implementation*. Berkeley: University of California Press.

Public Sector Consultants (PSC). 2011. "Final Report of Stakeholder Work Group Recommendations: Michigan Health Insurance Exchange Planning." June 17. Accessed July 12, 2013. http://www.mahp.org/federalreform/mahp/_Compilation%20of%20all%20final%20reports%206-17-11.pdf.

Purdum, Todd S. 2013. "The Obamacare Sabotage Campaign." *Politico*, November 1. Accessed February 24, 2014. http://www.politico.com/story/2013/11/the-obamacare-sabotage-campaign-99176.html.

Quick, Bob. 1994. "No More Raw Deal." *Santa Fe New Mexican*, January 26, D4. Accessed April 28, 2014. http://search.proquest.com/docview/331373716.

Rabe, Barry. 2011. "Contested Federalism and American Climate Policy." *Publius—The Journal of Federalism* 41 (3): 494–521.

Radnofsky, Louise, and Stephanie Armour. 2015. "State Officials Had Secret Huddle on Health-Law Subsidies." *Wall Street Journal*. June 1, 2015. Accessed September 30, 2015. http://www.wsj.com/articles/state-officials-had-secret-huddle-on-health-law-subsidies-1433202161.

Ragin, Charles. 1987. *The Comparative Method: Moving Beyond Qualitative and Quantitative Strategies*. Berkeley: University of California Press.

Regan, Priscilla M., and Christopher J. Deering. 2009. "State Opposition to REAL ID." *Publius* 39 (3): 476–505.

RetakeOurGov-Michigan PAC. 2011. "War Chest against SB 693 Senators." Retakeourgov.com. Accessed July 12, 2013. https://secure.piryx.com/donate/I4IyRYrJ/RetakeOurGov-Michigan/SB693.

Reynolds, Mark. 2012. "Legal Implications of Health Insurance Exchange Created by Executive Order." November 21. Letter. Accessed March 20, 2014. http://www.nmlegis.gov/lcs/handouts/LHHS%20091012%20Attorney%20General%20of%20NM%20Legal%20Implications%20of%20Health%20Insurance%20Exchange%20Created%20by%20Executive%20Order.pdf.

Rigby, Elizabeth, and Jake Haselswerdt. 2013. "Hybrid Federalism, Partisan Politics, and Early Implementation of State Health Insurance Exchanges." *Publius* 43 (3): 368–391.

Robert Wood Johnson Foundation (RWJF). 2011. "Fellow to Take on Health Care Reform for New Mexico." Accessed March 20, 2014. http://www.rwjf.org/en/about-rwjf/newsroom/newsroom-content/2011/12/fellow-to-take-on-health-care-reform-for-new-mexico.html.

Russell, Betsy Z. 2010. "'Health Freedom Act' Passes Idaho Senate." *The Spokesman-Review*, March 9. Accessed April 10, 2014. http://www.spokesman.com/stories/2010/mar/09/health-freedom-act-passes-idaho-senate/.

Russell, Betsy Z. 2012a. "Low Vote Turnout in Idaho Feared." *The Spokesman—Review*, May 6. Accessed April 12, 2014. http://www.spokesman.com/stories/2012/may/06/low-vote-turnout-feared/?print-friendly.

Russell, Betsy Z. 2012b. "Idaho Republicans Turn on One Another." *The Spokesman-Review*, May 8. Accessed April 12, 2014. http://www.spokesman.com/stories/2012/may/08/idaho-republicans-turn-one-another/.

Russell, Betsy Z. 2012c. "Denney, Moyle Use House Leadership PAC to Try to Defeat Roberts." *The Spokesman-Review*, May 8. Accessed April 12, 2014. http://www.spokesman.com/blogs/boise/2012/may/08/denney-moyle-use-house-leadership-pac-try-defeat-roberts/.

Russell, Betsy Z. 2013a. "Otter Facing Battles within GOP." *The Spokesman-Review*, January 6. Accessed April 12, 2014. http://www.spokesman.com/stories/2013/jan/06/otter-facing-battles-within-gop/.

Russell, Betsy Z. 2013b. "Testimony: 'Mr. Otter Now Owns Obamacare.'" *The Spokesman-Review*, February 7. Accessed April 28, 2014. http://www.spokesman.com/blogs/boise/2013/feb/07/testimony-mr-otter-now-owns-obamacare-keep-millions-idaho-liberty-jeopardy-law-land/.

Russell, Betsy Z. 2013c. "Senate Commerce Committee Votes 8-1 In Favor of Governor's Exchange Bill." *The Spokesman-Review*, February 7. Accessed April 28, 2014. http://www.spokesman.com/blogs/boise/2013/feb/07/senate-commerce-votes-8-1-favor-governors-exchange-bill/.

Russell, Betsy Z. 2013d. "Otter 'Grateful' For 8-1 Vote in Favor of His Health Exchange Bill." *The Spokesman-Review*, February 8. Accessed April 28, 2014. http://www.spokesman.com/blogs/boise/2013/feb/08/otter-grateful-8-1-vote-favor-his-health-exchange-bill/.

Russell, Betsy Z. 2013e. "Game Plan Shapes Up for Insurance Exchange Debate." *The Spokesman-Review*, February 19. Accessed April 28, 2014. http://www.spokesman.com/blogs/boise/2013/feb/19/game-plan-shapes-insurance-exchange-debate/.

Russell, Betsy Z. 2013f. "Idaho Senator Compares Health Exchange to Holocaust." *The Spokseman-Review*, January 30. Accessed April 28, 2014. http://www.spokesman.com/stories/2013/jan/30/idaho-senator-compares-health-exchange-holocaust/.

Russell, Betsey Z. 2013g. "Opponents Force Full Reading of Insurance Exchange Bill in the Senate." *The Spokesman-Review*, March 21. Accessed April 28, 2014. http://www.spokesman.com/blogs/boise/2013/mar/21/opponents-force-full-reading-insurance-exchange-bill-senate/.

Ryan, Paul. D. 2009. "The Patients' Choice Act: Summary." Accessed December 15, 2012. http://paulryan.house.gov/uploadedfiles/pcasummary15p.pdf.

Santelli, Rick. 2009. "Rick Santelli and 'Rant of the Year.'" User: Todd Sullivan. Accessed July 6, 2013. https://www.youtube.com/watch?v=bEZB4taSEoA.

Saltzman, Evan, and Christine Eibner. 2015. "The Effect of Eliminating the Affordable Care Acts Tax Credits in Federally Facilitated Marketplaces." The Rand Corporation. Accessed September 30, 2015. http://www.rand.org/content/dam/rand/pubs/research_reports/RR900/RR980/RAND_RR980.pdf.

Sarbaugh-Thomson, Marjorie *et al.* 2006. "Democracy among strangers: Term limits' effects on relationships between state legislators in Michigan." *State Politics and Policy Quarterly*. 6(4): 384–409.

Sebelius, Kathleen. 2013. "Letter to Governor Rick Snyder." March 5. Accessed July 12, 2013. http://www.cms.gov/CCIIO/Resources/Files/Downloads/mi-blueprint-letter-3-5-2013.pdf.

Shaffer, Stephen D and Dale Krane. 1992. *Mississippi Government and Politics: Modernizers versus Traditionalists*. Lincoln: University of Nebraska Press.

Shelly, Bryan. 2008. "Rebels and Their Causes: State Resistance to No Child Left Behind." *Publius—The Journal of Federalism* 38 (3): 444–468.

Shor, Boris. 2013. "ACA Implementation Votes in the States: Insurance Exchange, Medicaid Expansion, and Anti-Mandate Provisions." *Social Science Research Network*.

Shor, Boris, and Nolan McCarty. 2011. "The Ideological Mapping of American Legislatures." *American Political Science Review* 105 (3): 530–551.

Shiner, Meredith. 2009. "Haley Barbour: Health Care Reform like Jonestown." *Politico*, December 18. Accessed February 27. http://www.politico.com/news/stories/1209/30744.html.

Skocpol, Theda, and Vanessa Williamson. 2012. *The Tea Party and the Remaking of Republican Conservatism*. New York: Oxford University Press.

Skubick, Tim. 2012a. "One Reasonable GOP Legislator Sides with Gov. Snyder on Need for Marketplace Health Care Exchange." *MLive*. Accessed July 12, 2013. http://www.mlive.com/politics/index.ssf/2012/07/tim_skubick_one_reasonable_gop.html.

Skubick, Tim. 2012b. "Gov. Rick Snyder and Speaker Jase Bolger May Be On Collision Course." *MLive*. Accessed July 12, 2013. http://www.mlive.com/politics/index.ssf/2012/07/tim_skubick_gov_rick_snyder_an.html.

Snyder, Rick. 2011a. "Transcript of Rick Snyder's Inauguration Speech." *Detroit Free Press*. Accessed July 12, 2013. http://www.freep.com/article/20110101/NEWS15/110101024/Transcript-Rick-Snyder-s-inauguration-speech.

Snyder, Rick. 2011b. "A Special Message from Governor Rick Snyder: Health and Wellness." Accessed July 12, 2013. http://www.michigan.gov/snyder/0,4668,7-277--262254--,00.html

Snyder, Rick. 2012a. "Governor Issues Statement on Ruling of the Patient Protection and Affordable Care Act." Accessed July 12, 2013. http://www.michigan.gov/snyder/0,4668,7-277-57577_57657-281462--,00.html.

Snyder, Rick. 2012b. "Michigan Moves Toward State-Federal Partnership Health Exchange, Leaves Door Open for MI Health Marketplace." Accessed July 12, 2013. http://www.michigan.gov/snyder/0,4668,7-277-57577-290046--,00.html.

Snyder, Rick. 2013. "Letter to HHS Secretary Kathleen Sebelius." January 22. Accessed July 12, 2013. http://www.cms.gov/CCIIO/Resources/Technical-Implementation-Letters/Downloads/mi-marketplace-letter.pdf.

Somashekhar, Sandya. 2013. "Groups go Door-to-Door to Encourage Enrollment in Obamacare." *Washington Post*, August 2, 2013. Accessed September 30, 2015. https://www.washingtonpost.com/national/health-science/groups-go-door-to-door-to-encourage-enrollment-in-obamacare/2013/08/01/c6565c2c-f85a-11e2-afc1-c850c6ee5af8_story.html.

Sourcewatch. 2013. "Mackinac Center for Public Policy." Accessed July 12, 2013. http://www.sourcewatch.org/index.php/Mackinac_Center_for_Public_Policy.

Spangler, Todd. 2013. "Celebrating John Dingell, 'A True Man of the House.'" *Detroit Free Press*. Accessed July 6, 2013. http://www.freep.com/article/20130613/NEWS06/306130083/U-S-Rep-John-Dingell-feted-longest-serving-member-Congress.

Sparer, Michael S. 2011. "Federalism and the Patient Protection and Affordable Care Act of 2010: Why the Founding Fathers Would Not Be Surprised." *Journal of Health Politics Policy and Law* 36: 461–468.

Sparer, Michael S., and Lawrence D. Brown. 1996. "States and the Health Care Crisis: Limits and Lessons of Laboratory Federalism." In *Health Policy, Federalism, and the American States*, edited by R. F. Rich and W. D. White, 181–202. Washington, DC: Urban Institute Press.

Squire, Peverill. 2007. "Measuring State Legislative Professionalism: The Squire Index Revisited." *State Politics & Policy Quarterly*. 7(2): 211–227.

Starr, P. 2011. *Remedy and Reaction: The Peculiar American Struggle over Health Reform*. New Haven, CT: Yale University Press.

State Policy Network (SPN). 2013. "About SPN." Accessed July 12, 2013. http://www.spn.org/about/.

Steimel, Greg. 2013. "The Truth about the Mackinac Center." *Michigan Education Association*. Accessed July 13, 2013. http://www.mea.org/images/032513_The_Truth.pdf.

Stein, Sam. 2010. "Rep. Walt Minnick, Lone Dem Endorsed by Tea Party, Rejects Endorsed." *Huffington Post*, July 19. Accessed April 10, 2014. http://www.huffingtonpost.com/2010/07/19/rep-walt-minnick-lone-dem_n_651662.html.

Steinmo, Sven, and Jon Watts. 1995. "It's the Institutions Stupid! Why Comprehensive National Health Insurance Always Fails in America." *Journal of Health Politics, Policy and Law* 20 (2): 329–372.

Stiles, Andrew. 2013. "Obamacare and Its Cronies." *National Review Online*, December 3. http://www.nationalreview.com/article/365300/obamacare-and-its-cronies-andrew-stiles. Accessed February 24, 2014.

Stonecash, Jeffrey M. 1996. "The State Politics Literature: Moving beyond Covariation Studies and Pursuing Politics." *Polity* 28 (4): 559–579.

Tea Party 911. 2013. "Idaho Groups." Accessed April 10, 2014. http://www.teaparty911.com/info/locations/idaho.htm.

Tea Party Express. 2010. "Defeat Walt Minnick." Accessed April 28, 2014. http://www.teapartyexpress.org/251/defeat-walt-minnick-he-just-keeps-getting-more-and-more-liberal.

TheMSTeaParty. 2013. "MS Governor Phil Bryant Meeting with Leaders of MS Tea Party and Others." Retrieved from http://www.youtube.com/watch?v=uenXNl5YDCo.

Thoms, Sue. 2011. "Gov. Rick Snyder Unveils Plan to Make Michigan Residents Healthier." Accessed July 12, 2013. *MLive*.http://www.mlive.com/health/index.ssf/2011/09/snyder_unveils_plan_to_get_mic.html.

Thoms, Sue. 2012. "Michigan Reacts: Quotes about Supreme Court Ruling on Affordable Care Act." *MLive*. Accessed July 12, 2013. http://www.mlive.com/news/index.ssf/2012/06/michigan_reacts_key_quotes_abo.html.

Toobin, Jeffrey. 2015. "Doom for a Cynical Assault on Obamacare." *New Yorker*. June 25, 2015. Accessed September 30, 2015. http://www.newyorker.com/news/daily-comment/doom-for-a-cynical-assault-on-obamacare.

Tumulty, Karen, Kate Pickert, and Alice Park. 2010. "America's New Prescription." *Time Magazine*. Accessed September 30, 2015. http://content.time.com/time/specials/packages/article/0,28804,1975068_1975012_1974994,00.html.

Warwick, Tricia. 2013. "New Mexico Health Insurance Exchange Inaugural Board Meeting." Accessed March 20, 2014. http://www.nmhix.com/wp-content/uploads/2013/05/ApprovedMinutesForInauguralMeeting_4-29-2013.pdf.

United Press International (UPI). 2011. "Mich. Governor Recall Effort Appears Weak." *United Press International*. Accessed July 12, 2013. http://www.upi.com/Top_News/US/2011/07/03/Mich-governor-recall-effort-appears-weak/UPI-84231309744195/.

United States House Roll Call #165. 2010. "Final Vote Results for Roll Call 165." Accessed March 14, 2014. http://clerk.house.gov/evs/2010/roll165.xml.

United States Senate Vote #396. 2010. "HR 3590 (111th): Patient Protection and Affordable Care Act." Accessed April 28, 2014. https://www.govtrack.us/congress/votes/111-2009/s396.

Vestal, Christine. 2012. "States Get More Time to Decide if They Will Run Their Own Exchanges." *Pew States*. Accessed April 28, 2014. http://www.pewstates.org/projects/stateline/headlines/states-get-more-time-to-decide-if-they-will-run-their-own-health-insurance-exchanges-85899430743.

Volden, Craig. 2005. "Intergovernmental Political Competition in American Federalism." *American Journal of Political Science* 49: 327–342.

Weissert, W. G., and C. S. Weissert. 2012. *Governing Health: The Politics of Health Policy*. Baltimore, MD: Johns Hopkins University Press.

Werner, Erica. 2010. "Obama Prefers a National Health Insurance Exchange, Siding with House over Senate." *Associated Press*, January 12. Accessed April 2, 2013. http://www.cleveland.com/nation/index.ssf/2010/01/obama_prefers_a_national_healt.html.

Whitaker, Morgan. 2013. "Mississippi Lawmakers Save Medicaid, but GOP Blocks Expansion." *MSNBC*. Accessed April 28, 2014. http://www.msnbc.com/politicsnation/mississippi-lawmakers-save-medicaid-gop.

White, Jennifer, Mercedes Mejia, and Zoe Clark. 2012. "Michigan Attorney General Bill Schuette Urges Delay in Creating Health Care Exchanges." *Michigan Radio*. Accessed July 12, 2013. http://www.michiganradio.org/post/michigan-attorney-general-bill-schuette-urges-delay-creating-health-care-exchanges

White House. 2010. "Remarks by the President and Vice-President at Signing of the Health Insurance Reform Bill." Accessed December 15, 2012. http://www.whitehouse.gov/the-press-office/remarks-president-and-vice-president-signing-health-insurance-reform-bill.

White House. 2012. "2012 Progress Report: States are Implementing Health Reform." Accessed March 2, 2014. http://www.whitehouse.gov/sites/default/files/01-18-12_exchange_report.pdf.

Williams, Jim. 2011. "Martinez Vetoes Bills for State Tax Credits, Health Insurance Exchange, and Define Autism in School." *KUNM*, April 8. Accessed March 14, 2014. http://m.kunm.org/?utm_referrer=#mobile/1818.

Wright, Samantha. 2012. "Idaho Primary: Why the GOP Closed Its Ballot." *Boise State Public Radio*, May 9. Accessed April 11, 2014. http://boisestatepublicradio.org/post/idaho-primary-why-gop-closed-its-ballot.

Yackee, Susan, and Jason Webb Yackee. 2009. "Divided Government and U.S. Federal Rulemaking." *Regulation and Governance* 3 (2): 128–144.

Yetter, Deborah. 2016. "Beshear Group Rips Bevin over Benefit System." *The Courrier-Journal*, April 4, 2016. Accessed September 28, 2016. http://www.courier-journal.com/story/news/politics/2016/04/04/beshear-group-rips-bevin-over-benefit-system/82611344/.

Young, Jeffrey. 2012. "Republican Governors Ask for Meeting with President, Obamacare Deadline Extension." *Huffington Post*, November 15. Accessed March 2, 2014. http://www.huffingtonpost.com/2012/11/14/governors-obamacare_n_2132080.html.

INDEX

The manufacturer's authorised representative in the EU for product
safety is Oxford University Press España S.A. of El Parque Empresarial
San Fernando de Henares, Avenida de Castilla, 2 - 28830 Madrid
(www.oup.es/en or product.safety@oup.com). OUP España S.A. also acts
as importer into Spain of products made by the manufacturer.
Printed and bound by CPI Group (UK) Ltd, Croydon, CR0 4YY
14/09/2026
02216305-0019